Anti-Cancer Smoothies

Quick and easy delicious smoothie recipes to a healthy you

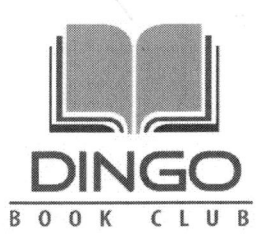

DINGO
BOOK CLUB

"Great Books Change Life"

© Copyright 2018 by Dingo Publishing - All rights reserved.

The contents of this book may not be reproduced, duplicated or transmitted without direct written permission from the author.

Under no circumstances will any legal responsibility or blame be held against the publisher for any reparation, damages, or monetary loss due to the information herein, either directly or indirectly.

Legal Notice:

This book is copyright protected. This is only for personal use. You cannot amend, distribute, sell, use, quote or paraphrase any part or the content within this book without the consent of the author.

Disclaimer Notice:

Please note the information contained within this document is for educational and entertainment purposes only. Every attempt has been made to provide accurate, up to date and reliable complete information. No warranties of any kind are expressed or implied. Readers acknowledge that the author is not engaging in the rendering of legal, financial, medical or professional advice. The content of this book has been derived from various sources. Please consult a licensed professional before attempting any techniques outlined in this book.

By reading this document, the reader agrees that under no circumstances is the author responsible for any losses, direct or indirect, which are incurred as a result of the use of information contained within this document, including, but not limited to, — errors, omissions, or inaccuracies.

Introduction 8

Chapter 1: Anti-Cancer Nutrition 10

    Difficulties faced by cancer patients 12

    Importance of Nutrients 13

    Anti-cancer diet guidelines 16

Chapter 2: Anti-Cancer Smoothie Recipes 21

    1. Anti-Cancer Breakfast Smoothie 21

    2. Strawberry Breakfast Smoothie 23

    3. Berry Chocolate Cancer Fighting Smoothie 25

    4. Carrot-Mango Green Tea Smoothie 26

    5. Green Cleansing Smoothie 27

    6. Spring Detox Smoothie 29

    7. Artichoke Smoothie 30

    8. Kale, Banana and Seeds Super food Smoothie 32

    9. Nectarine, Mixed Berry and Coconut Smoothie 33

    10. Strawberry Hemp Seed Smoothie 34

    11. Banana Smoothie with Nuts and Seeds 35

    12. Pumpkin Spice Latte Smoothie 36

    13. Raspberry Anti-Cancer Smoothie 37

    14. Very Berry Antioxidant Smoothie 38

    15. Berry Overload Smoothie 39

    16. Vegetable Blast 40

    17. Fruit and Vegetable Smoothie 41

    18. Red Smoothie 42

19. Roasted Vegetable Smoothie 44
20. Spicy Anti-Inflammatory Smoothie 46
21. Grapefruit Berry Mint 47
22. Papaya Guava Smoothie 48
23. Loaded Anti-oxidant Smoothie 49
24. Watermelon Smoothie 50
25. Pumpkin Smoothie 51
26. Sweet Potato Smoothie 52
27. Strawberry Apple Smoothie 53
28. Garlic Veggie Smoothie 54
29. Berry Flaxseed and Pomegranate Smoothie 55
30. Rosemary Green Smoothie 56
31. Spicy Tomato Smoothie 57
32. Veggie Smoothie 58
33. Anti-inflammatory Green Smoothie 59
34. Pumpkin Cranberry Smoothie 60
35. Apple and Spinach Smoothie 61
36. Cancer Killer Smoothie 62
37. Fruit Salad Smoothie 63
38. Cooling Watermelon Smoothie 64
39. Immune Boosting Graviola Super Smoothie 65
40. Maca Smoothie 66
41. Super Smoothie 67
42. Chai Blackberry Smoothie 68

Chapter 3: Anti-Cancer Smoothie Bowl Recipes 69

1. Butternut, Carrot & Turmeric Smoothie Bowl 69
2. Enlighten Smoothie Bowl 71
3. Black Forest Smoothie Bowl.....................................73
4. Tropical Smoothie Bowl..75
5. Chocolate Hazelnut Hemp Smoothie Bowl.............76
6. Raspberry Almond Butter Smoothie Bowl.............77
7. Cream n Strawberry Smoothie Bowl 78
8. Red Berry Smoothie Bowl...79
9. Kale and Avocado Smoothie Bowl 81
10. Pineapple, Peach and Banana Smoothie Bowl........ 82
11. Dark Cherry Smoothie Bowl................................... 83
12. Mixed Berry Smoothie Bowl.................................... 84
13. Green Smoothie Bowl 85
14. Peach, Orange, and Berry Smoothie Bowl 87
15. Super Food Avocado Smoothie Bowl with Cashew Cream 88
16. Pitaya Breakfast Bowl 90
17. Peach-Raspberry Smoothie Bowl........................... 91

Chapter 4: Anti-Cancer Layered Smoothie Recipes 92

1. Two layered Mango – Peach and Strawberry – Banana Smoothie..92
2. Tropical Layered Smoothie 94
3. Sunrise Smoothie 96
4. Super Healthy Rainbow Smoothie...........................97

5. Avocado Strawberry Layered Smoothie 100
6. Berry Beet Smoothie 102
7. Cherry Mango Smoothie..104
8. Hawaiian Berry Smoothie..105
9. Layered Mixed Berry Green Power Smoothie........106
10. Strawberry Mango Smoothie................................. 108
11. Berry, Banana and Kale Smoothie 109
12. Multi-layered Smoothie 111
13. Chocolate, Banana and Pumpkin Swirl Super Smoothie 113

Chapter 5: Anti-Cancer Dessert Smoothies........... 114

1. Roasted Strawberry Smoothie................................ 114
2. Dreamy Strawberry Smoothie Layered with Chia Seed Pudding 116
3. Banana Bread Smoothie 118
4. Kiwi Berry Mousse Smoothie 119
5. Apple Pie Smoothie 121
6. Fruit Cake Smoothie 122
7. Pumpkin Pie Smoothie 123
8. Peanut Butter and Oatmeal Smoothie 124
9. Strawberry Cheesecake Smoothie 125
10. Brownie Smoothie 126
11. Super Food Pumpkin Pie Green Smoothie............127
12. Chocolate Oatmeal Cookie Smoothie..................128
13. Carrot Cake Smoothie 129

14.	Chocolate Peanut Butter Smoothie	130
15.	Triple Berry Kefir Smoothie	131
16.	Red Velvet Green Smoothie	132
17.	Blueberry Cheesecake Smoothie	133

Conclusion **134**

Bonus **135**

More books from us **137**

Introduction

I want to thank you for purchasing this book, '*Anti-cancer smoothies*' and hope you find the content informative and useful.

You will find a wide range of books on anti-cancer diets when you walk by the health section of any bookstore. Why is there a sudden awareness on anti-cancer diets? Well, it is because one in 25 Americans is diagnosed with Cancer or defined as a Cancer survivor. The trend to turn to healthy and organic vegetables, fruit and greens has now become a necessity.

Irrespective of whether you have cancer or are at risk of getting cancer due to your genes, your food habits play a big role on your health. The right food gives your body the ability to battle the disease or curb it once and for all. The conventional treatment given to cancer patients can cause a series of side effects that can damage certain other organs in the body or destroy a few healthy cells. Therefore, the body will need a lot of nutrients, minerals, vitamins and fats to maintain any kind of quality of life.

The best strategy to get your body back to its healthy functioning mode or reduce the risk of cancer attack is by following the anti-cancer diet. According to the American Cancer Society, a person should eat a minimum of five portions of vegetables and fruit daily along with their regular diet. Medical experts and researchers have found that certain foods can prevent the risk of cancer. It is, therefore, a good idea to start including cancer-fighting foods in your diet to help reduce the risk.

The Anti-cancer smoothie recipes in the book are made from vegetables, spices, fruit and herbs, which help fight cancer. They are said to provide the required nutrients to boost your body's immune system. A few recipes also help to detox your body, make you feel lighter and more energetic.

I hope this book serves as an informative and interesting read to you!

Happy Reading!

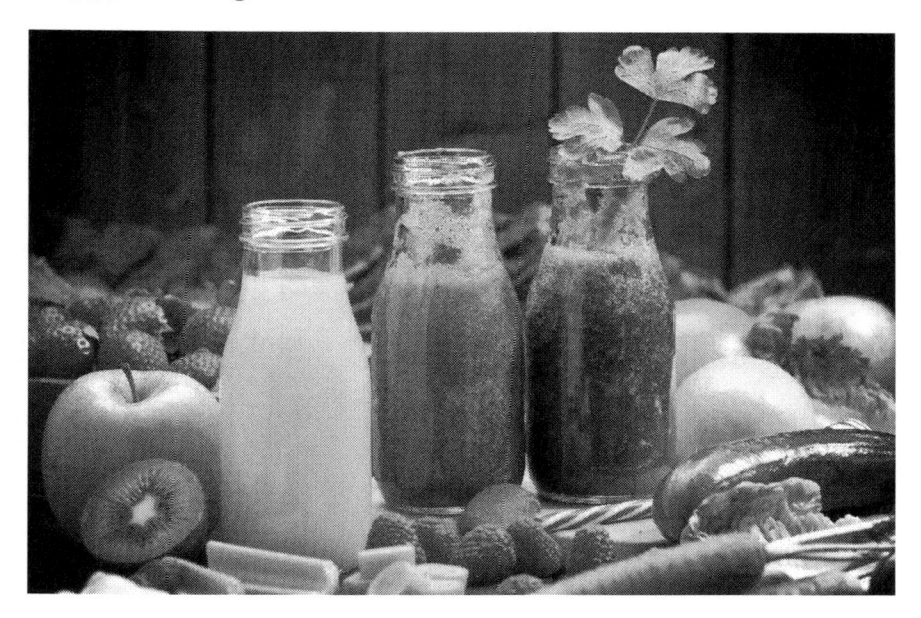

Chapter 1: Anti-Cancer Nutrition

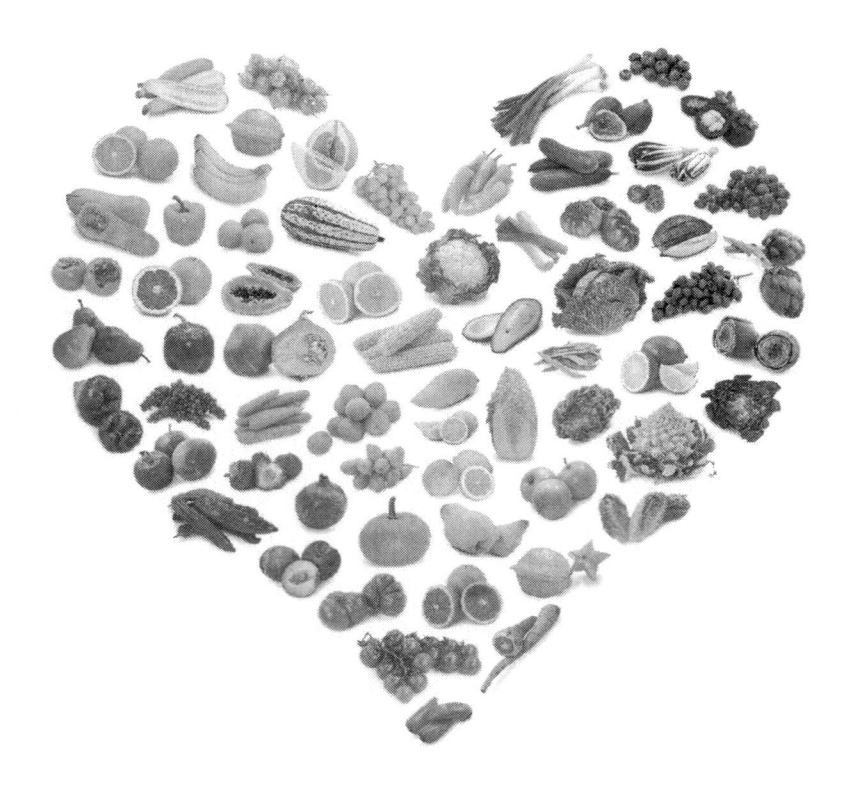

Nutrition is required to keep your body healthy – the food we consume provides the nutrition necessary for the growth of bones and the tissue replacement process. Your body needs the right kind of food to stay hale and healthy. Eating foods that have all the required nutrients such as proteins, minerals, carbohydrates, vitamins and fat helps the body perform its required functionality.

One of the biggest, or perhaps the biggest, health threat to people across the world is cancer. In the past few decades, cancer has taken the lives of millions. More often than not, cancer cannot be treated completely; you can just fight it until it rebounds. The good news is cancer-fighting foods can help reduce the risk of cancer.

Providing the right nutrition to the body before and after the cancer treatment can help cancer survivors feel better. Cancer and its treatment cause severe side effects to the body and weakens the immune system. Proper food and right nutrition can help to improve their quality of life. Nutrition therapy can help cancer survivors to maintain healthy body weight, keep the bones and tissues strong and reduce the side effects of cancer drugs. Most people find it difficult to eat when they are going through cancer treatments. The following cancer treatments can affect the nutrition of the body:

- Surgery
- Chemotherapy
- Stem cell transplantation
- Hormone therapy
- Immunotherapy
- Radiation therapy

It is tough for the body to absorb nutrients when the cancer treatment affects the stomach, pancreas, intestines, liver, head, esophagus or neck.

Difficulties faced by cancer patients

Most cancer treatments also affect the ability to consume enough food required for the body. These treatments influence the smell, taste, appetite or the potential to absorb the necessary nutrients from the food eaten. This can result in malnutrition (lack of major nutrients). Malnutrition can cause weakness and weariness in patients. The body will not be able to tackle foreign bodies or fight infection. This might also take the patient to a stage where he will not be able to complete the cancer treatment, as his body will not have the strength to tolerate the high doses of drugs or therapies. If the cancer spreads or grows, then it worsens the patient's condition.

Cachexia and Anorexia are the types of malnutrition found in cancer patients. What is Cachexia? It is a condition caused by weight loss (weakness), loss of fat and muscle loss. This is most common with patients affected by tumors, as they have problems with digestion or cannot eat properly. Some patients eat well, but the nutrients in the food don't get stored in the body as fat or muscle, as the tumor cells absorb all the nutrients, resulting in tumor growth. These tumors modify the way the body uses specific nutrients. For instance, a tumor growth in the neck, intestines, head or stomach uses the protein, carbohydrates and fat from the body to increase the growth of cancerous cells (in the tumor area). Though the patient eats enough food, the body will not be able to absorb the required nutrients from the food as the tumor alters the course of the process.

What is Anorexia? It is the condition caused when the patient loses his appetite or is not interested in food. This is a common symptom in almost all cancer patients. Anorexia can occur during the initial or later stages of cancer – especially when cancer grows or spreads.

Some cancer patients can have both cachexia and anorexia at the same time.

Importance of Nutrients

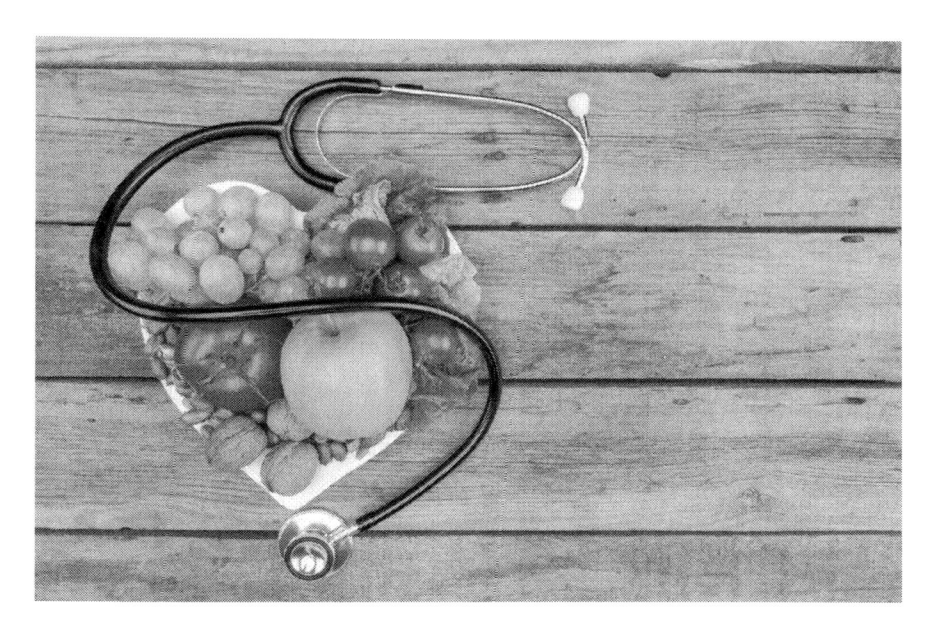

Though including cancer-fighting foods into your diet cannot completely guarantee cancer prevention, the right choices can definitely reduce its risk. The American Cancer Society asked a group of nutritional experts and cancer specialists to come up with proper anti-cancer diet plans to help people. These experts and specialists have been stressing the importance of choosing a diet that is rich in whole grains, vegetables and fruit.

The findings and evidence highlight that every individual should consume 1 ½ to 2 cups of fruit and 2 to 3 cups of vegetables regularly. The anti cancer diet is high in phytochemicals, vitamins and minerals but low in calories. If you are planning to consume fruit in the form of juices, it is advisable to have cold-pressed juices (whole fruit) with no sugar or sweetener.

Whole grains are loaded with antioxidant and anti-cancer compounds. According to experts, a person should consume a minimum of three one-ounce portions of whole grains in a day. One serving is a half-cup of brown rice, oatmeal or whole-grain bread or pasta.

The high fiber content in these foods will make you feel full even when consumed in smaller portions. In case of obesity, it is necessary to limit the consumption of beverages and high-calorie foods to help in weight loss. All processed food, fried food, fast food or oily junk food falls under this category. Irrespective of your body weight, eating these high-calorie foods (even in small proportions) might cause inflammatory issues.

It is crucial to maintain a healthy body weight to ward off cancerous cells or tumor cells. How do you know if you have a healthy body weight? Checking the body mass index or BMI can help determine if you have the right body weight. Most dieticians and clinicians use BMI to determine if a person has healthy body weight or not.

If the BMI is,

- Greater than 25, the body is considered to be overweight
- Greater than 30, the person is obese

If you fall in either of these categories, it is high time to make changes in your lifestyle, food habits and sleep routines. The most important of all is to manage your stress and keep it under control.

Apart from these, your body requires the following:

- 2.5 hours of moderate physical activity per week
- More than six hours of sleep (at night) regularly
- Enough time to relax and to reduce your stress levels
- Complete rest to your body once a week

Anti-cancer diet guidelines

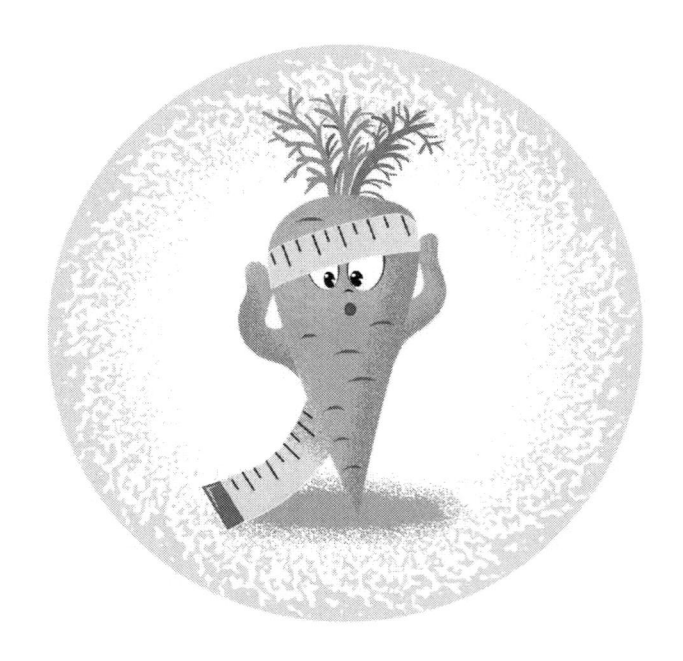

Studies have shown that high intake of fruit, vegetables, fiber and foods rich in calcium helps to reduce the risk of lung, colorectal and breast cancers. These foods are termed as cancer-fighting foods. Unhealthy BMI (body mass index), consumption of processed and red meat, abdominal obesity and regular alcohol intake resulted in increased risk of the deadly disease (cancer).

Following these guidelines on the anti-cancer diet may help to reduce the risk of cancer or to manage the disease to an extent.

Include plenty of vegetables and fruit in your diet

Vegetables and fruit are high in minerals and vitamins that can reduce the risk of certain types of cancer. Eating more plant-based food encourages your body to control the cravings for sugar and other high-calorie foods. Eat more fruit or vegetable salads instead of filling your stomach with cakes, pastries, oily snacks, etc. Say no to sugary or processed or junk foods! Try the Mediterranean diet, as it usually comprises of items that are rich in cancer-fighting nutrients as they focus mostly on plant-based foods. Their diet is full of legumes, whole grains, vegetables, fruit and nuts. The meal is either topped or cooked with olive oil.

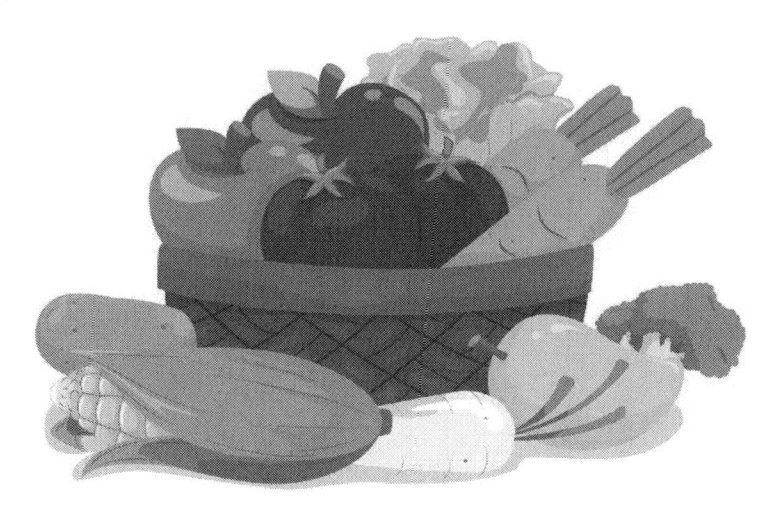

Drink more green tea everyday

Green tea is considered an important part of the anti-cancer diet because of its rich antioxidant property. It is helpful in preventing lung, breast, pancreatic, liver, skin and esophageal cancer. According to researchers; epigallocatechin-3 gallate, a non-toxic chemical found in green tea, works against urokinase, the enzyme which is crucial for the growth of cancer. A cup of green tea has around 100 to 200 milligrams (mg) of epigallocatechin-3 gallate.

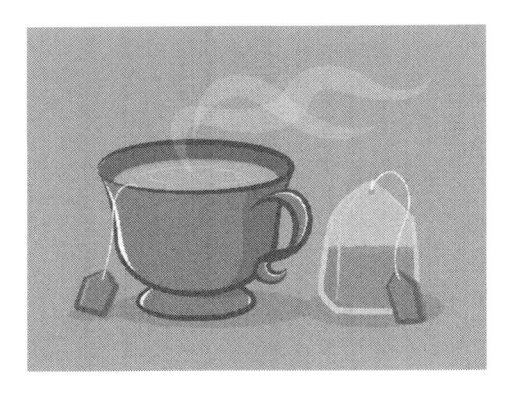

More tomatoes can help

Studies and researches have confirmed that lycopene, an antioxidant found in tomatoes is more influential than vitamin E, beta-carotene, and alpha-carotene. The antioxidant (lycopene) is an anti-cancer food that helps to protect the body against certain types of cancer such as lung and prostate cancer. When you cook the tomatoes, the lycopene in the vegetable gets released and made available to your body.

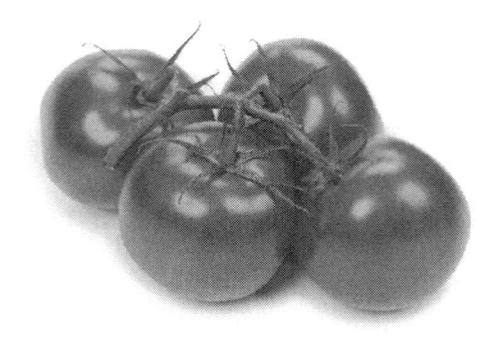

Olive oil is the best

Olive oil has mono-unsaturated fat, which makes it an excellent cancer-fighting food. People in Mediterranean countries use olive oil for cooking and also as dressing oil. Studies have shown that breast cancer rates are fifty percent less in Mediterranean nations when compared to the United States.

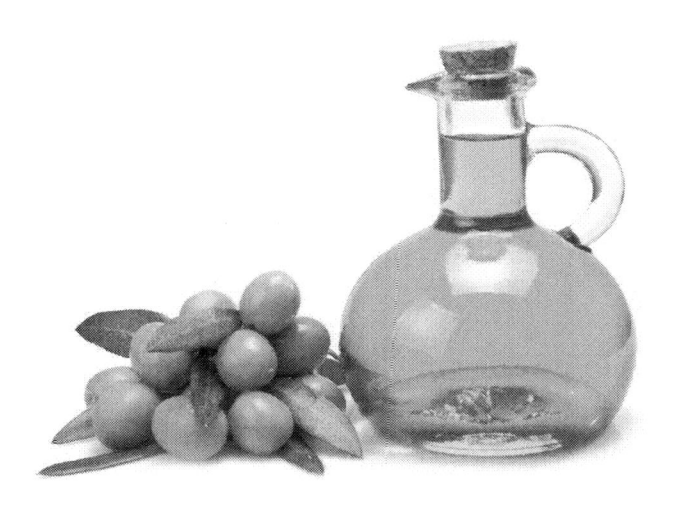

Grapes can make a healthy snack

The seeds of red grapes have the super antioxidant, Activin, which is an excellent cancer-fighting chemical. Activin is also found in grape juice (made from red grapes) and red wine. This compound might offer major protection against chronic degenerative diseases, heart conditions and certain types of cancer.

Add more onions and garlic to your food

The nutrients in onions and garlic can stop the development of nitrosamines (potent carcinogens) that target several organs, such as breasts, colon and liver. Onions and garlic will have more sulfur compounds when they are more pungent. The sulfur content in these vegetables can prevent cancer.

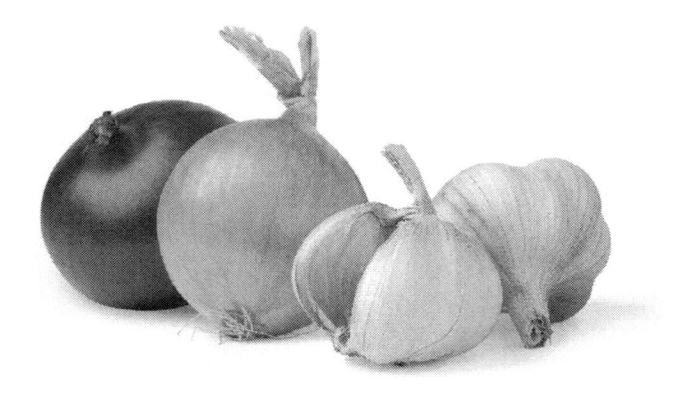

Try to include as much nutritious food as possible into your diet to prevent cancer from crawling into your body.

Chapter 2: Anti-Cancer Smoothie Recipes

1. Anti-Cancer Breakfast Smoothie

Serves: 1 large glass or 2 smaller glasses

Ingredients:

- 1 small ripe banana, peeled and sliced
- 2 tablespoons hemp seeds
- 1 ½ cups filtered water
- ¼ cup pomegranate arils, fresh or frozen
- ½ cup frozen strawberries
- 2 cups fresh salad greens or spinach or collard greens or lightly steamed kale
- 1 tablespoon cocoa powder, unsweetened
- ½ tablespoon ground chia seeds
- Juice of ½ lime
- ½ inch knob fresh ginger
- A handful fresh mint leaves
- 1 tablespoon flax meal
- ¼ cup frozen raw broccoli florets

Method:

2. Add the hemp seeds and water into the blender.
3. Blend on high speed for 15 seconds.

4. Add banana, pomegranate and strawberries and blend for another 15 seconds.
5. Add salad greens, cocoa, chia seeds, lime juice, ginger, mint leaves, flax meal and broccoli into the blender.
6. Blend for 30 -40 seconds or until smooth.
7. Pour into a large glass or into 2 smaller glasses.
8. Serve immediately.

2. Strawberry Breakfast Smoothie

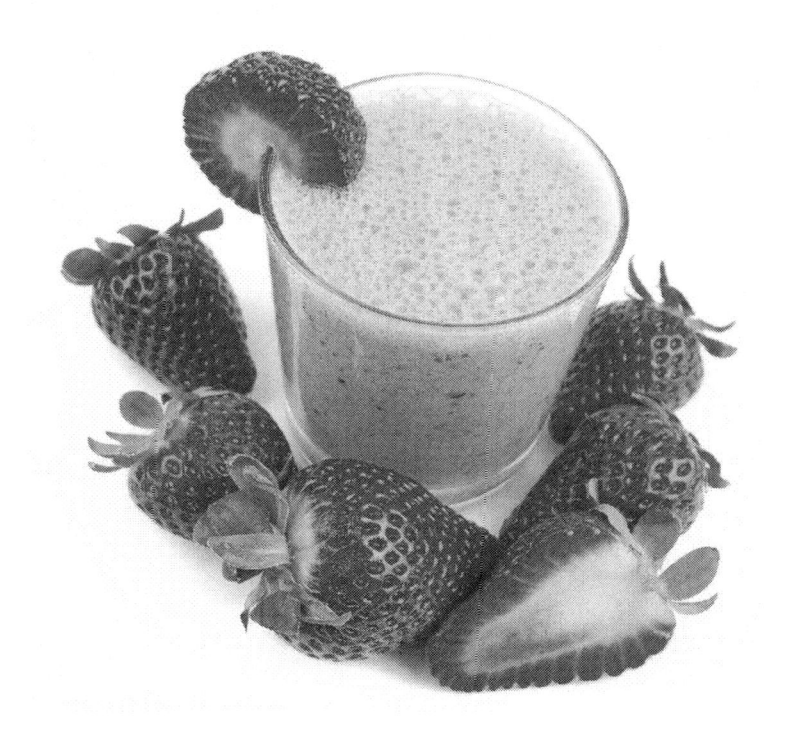

Ingredients:

- 2 cups spinach, chopped
- 10 strawberries, hulled and sliced
- 2 whole strawberries for garnish
- 2 cups soy milk
- 2/3 cup cooked oats
- Honey or agave nectar (optional)
- ½ cup plain Greek yogurt
- 2 tablespoons chia seeds

Method:

1. Add milk, strawberries, oats, honey, spinach, yogurt and chia seeds into a blender. Blend for 30-40 seconds or until smooth.
2. Pour into tall glasses. Garnish with slices of strawberry and serve with crushed ice.

3. Berry Chocolate Cancer Fighting Smoothie

Ingredients:

- 1 small banana, sliced
- 1/8 avocado, cut into small pieces
- 3-4 baby carrots, diced
- ½ cup kale leaves, fresh or frozen
- 1 tablespoon raw cacao powder or cocoa powder, unsweetened
- Water, as required
- ¾ cup frozen strawberries
- ½ cup destemmed kale leaves, fresh or frozen
- ½ tablespoon flaxseeds
- 5-6 raisins
- ½ scoop protein powder (optional)
- Ice cubes, as required

Method:

1. Add banana, avocado, carrots, cocoa, kale leaves, water, strawberries, flaxseeds, raisins, protein powder and ice cubes into a blender.
2. Blend for 40-50 seconds or until smooth.
3. Pour into a tall glass.
4. Serve immediately.

4. Carrot-Mango Green Tea Smoothie

Ingredients:

- ½ cup carrots, peeled and sliced
- ½ inch fresh ginger, peeled and sliced
- 1 ½ cups water
- 1 cup frozen mango chunks
- 2 green tea bags
- ½ teaspoon honey or to taste
- ½ tablespoon chia seeds (optional)

Method:

1. Add water into a saucepan. Place the saucepan over medium heat.
2. When water begins to boil, add carrots and cook until tender.
3. Add ginger and cook for 2 more minutes and turn off the heat.
4. Drop the tea bags in it. Cover the saucepan with a lid. Uncover and remove the tea bags. Squeeze the tea bags to remove as much liquid as possible.
5. Discard the tea bags and ginger slices. Cool and chill for 10 minutes.
6. Add carrot- green tea mixture into the blender.
7. Add mango, chia seeds and honey.
8. Blend for 30-40 seconds or until smooth.
9. Pour into tall glasses and serve immediately.

5. Green Cleansing Smoothie

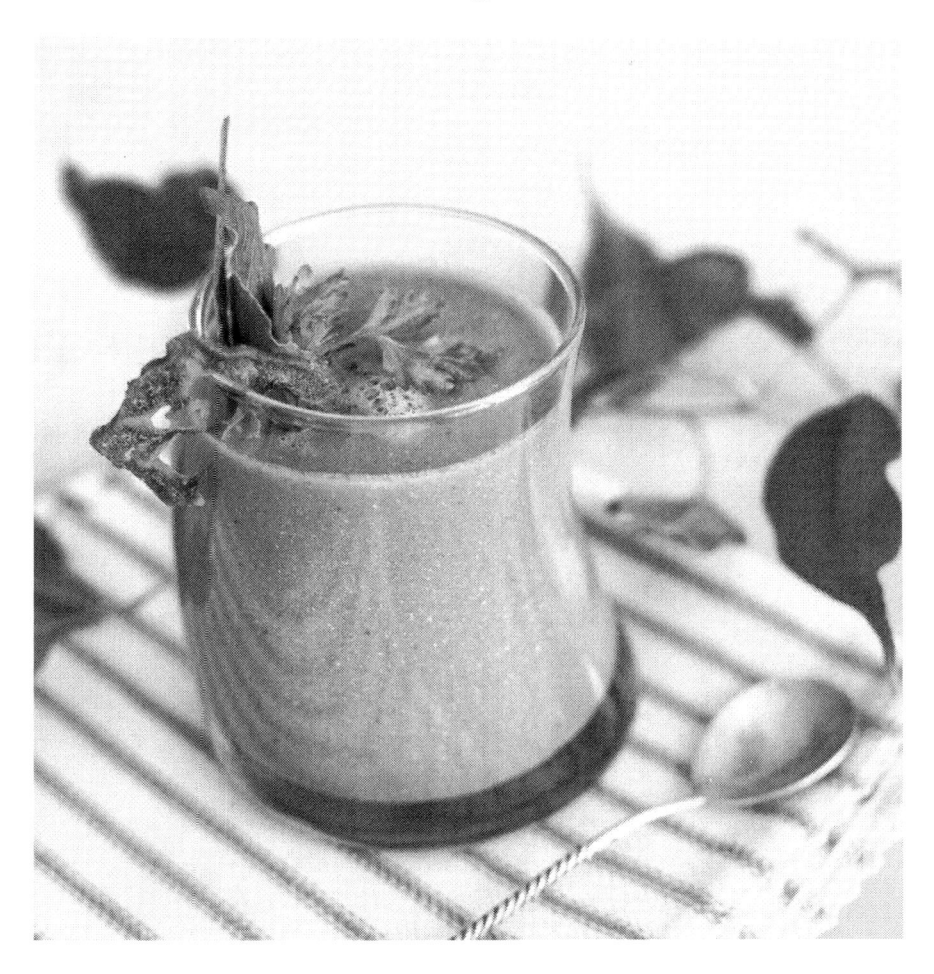

Ingredients:

- 2 bananas, peel, slice and freeze
- 1 cup spinach, chopped
- 1 cup kale leaves, chopped
- 1 cup celery
- 2 cups romaine lettuce, chopped

- 1 small cucumber, chopped
- 1 large red apple, cored and chopped
- A handful fresh parsley
- A handful mint leaves
- ½ inch piece fresh ginger, sliced
- 1 teaspoon ground cinnamon (optional)
- 1 tablespoon lemon juice
- 1 teaspoon chia seeds
- ¼ teaspoon turmeric powder
- A pinch cayenne pepper (optional)
- Natural sweetener like stevia or honey (optional - to taste)
- 2 cups coconut water

Method:

1. Add bananas, spinach, kale, celery, lettuce, cucumber, apple, parsley, mint, ginger, cinnamon, lemon juice, chia seeds, turmeric powder, coconut water, cayenne pepper and sweetener (optional) into a blender.
2. Blend for 30-40 seconds or until smooth.
3. Add coconut water and adjust as per the consistency you prefer.
4. Pour into tall glasses and serve with crushed ice.

6. Spring Detox Smoothie

Ingredients:

- 1 avocado, peeled and chopped
- 2 cups baby kale or any other greens of your choice
- 2 cups pineapple chunks
- 2 cups cucumber
- Juice of 2 lemons
- 2 cups cilantro
- 2 tablespoons freshly grated ginger
- 2 cups green tea, chilled

Method:

1. Add kale, pineapple cilantro, cucumber, lemon juice, avocado slices, ginger and green tea into a blender.
2. Blend for 30-40 seconds or until smooth.
3. Add water if you like a smoothie of thinner consistency.
4. Pour into tall glasses and serve with crushed ice.

7. Artichoke Smoothie

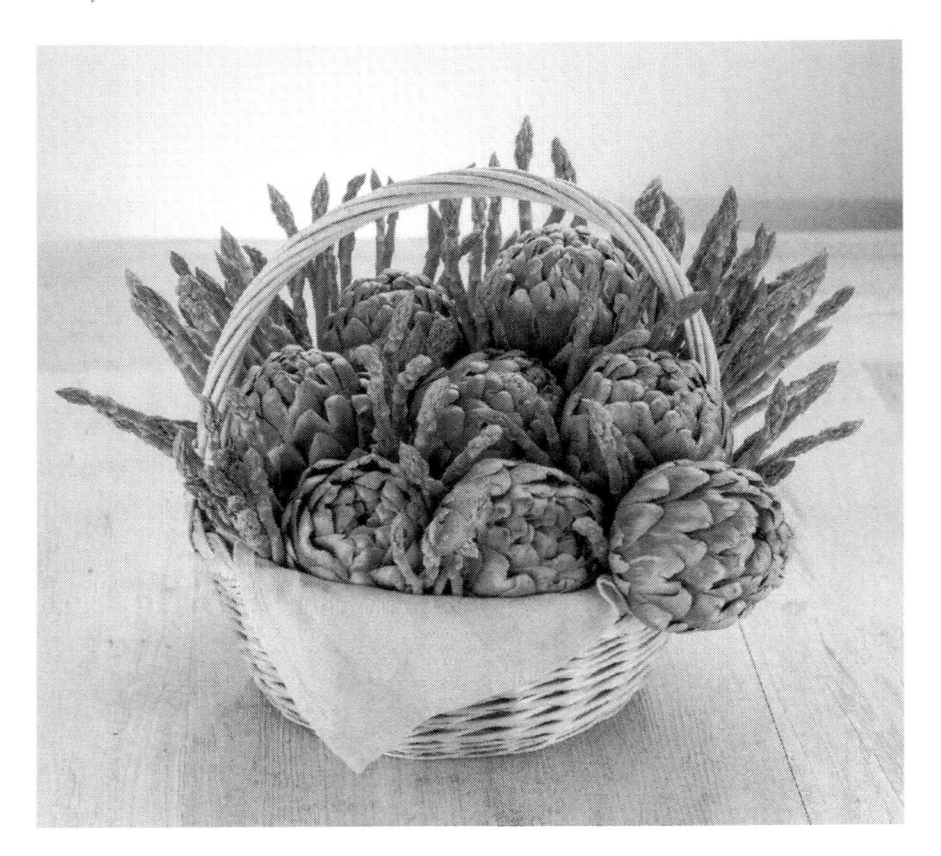

Ingredients:

- 2 apples, sliced
- 2 cups artichokes, chopped
- 1 inch ginger, peeled and sliced
- 2 cloves garlic, peeled
- ½ cup fresh cilantro
- ½ cup fresh parsley
- 6 -8 baby carrots
- ½ cup water

Method:

1. Add apples, artichokes, ginger, garlic, cilantro, parsley, baby carrots and water into a blender.
2. Blend for 30-40 seconds or until smooth.
3. Add more water if you like a smoothie of thinner consistency.
4. Pour into tall glasses and serve with crushed ice.

8. Kale, Banana and Seeds Super food Smoothie

Ingredients:

- 1 ripe medium banana, peeled and sliced
- 1 ½ cups almond milk
- 2 tablespoons raw shelled hemp seeds
- 1 tablespoon chia seeds
- 2 cups ice cubes
- 2 dates, pitted
- 1 ½ cups baby kale

Method:

1. Add almond milk, hemp seeds, chia seeds, ice cubes, dates, banana and kale into a blender.
2. Blend for 30-40 seconds or until smooth.
3. Add more almond milk if you like a smoothie of thinner consistency.
4. Pour into tall glasses and serve.

9. Nectarine, Mixed Berry and Coconut Smoothie

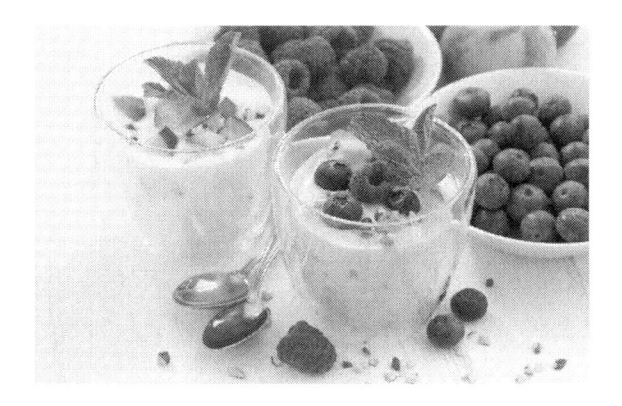

Ingredients:

- 2 medium nectarines, peeled and chopped
- 1 cup coconut water
- ¼ cup frozen strawberries
- ¼ cup frozen blueberries
- ¼ cup frozen raspberries
- ¼ cup frozen blackberries

Method:

1. Add coconut water, all the berries and nectarines into a blender.
2. Blend for 30-40 seconds or until smooth. Add more coconut water if you like a smoothie of thinner consistency.
3. Pour into tall glasses and serve.

10. Strawberry Hemp Seed Smoothie

Ingredients:

- 2 cups milk of your choice
- 2 cups frozen strawberries
- 1 cup frozen raspberries
- ½ cup frozen blackberries
- ½ cup frozen blueberries
- ½ cup hemp seeds
- 2 cups vanilla yogurt
- 2 teaspoons vanilla extract
- 6-8 dates, pitted (optional)

Method:

1. Add milk, all the berries, hemp seeds, vanilla yogurt, vanilla extract and dates into a blender.
2. Blend for 30-40 seconds or until smooth.
3. Add more almond milk if you like a smoothie of thinner consistency.
4. Pour into tall glasses and serve.

11. Banana Smoothie with Nuts and Seeds

Ingredients:

- 2 ripe bananas, peeled and sliced
- 2 tablespoons sunflower seeds
- 2 tablespoons pumpkin seeds
- 2 tablespoons flaxseeds
- 16 almonds
- 2 cups almond milk
- ¼ teaspoon ground turmeric
- 4 teaspoons almond butter
- ½ teaspoon vanilla extract
- 2 teaspoons honey
- Ice cubes, as required
- Freshly ground nutmeg, to sprinkle on top

Method:

1. Add banana, all the seeds, almonds, almond milk, turmeric powder, almond butter, vanilla extract, honey and ice cubes into a blender.
2. Blend for 30-40 seconds or until smooth.
3. Add more almond milk if you like a smoothie of thinner consistency.
4. Pour into tall glasses.
5. Sprinkle nutmeg on top and serve.

12. Pumpkin Spice Latte Smoothie

Ingredients:

- 2 bananas, peeled and sliced
- 2 cups almond milk or any other milk of your choice, unsweetened
- 4 teaspoons pumpkin pie spice
- 1 cup canned pumpkin
- 4 teaspoons maple syrup
- ½ cup ice cubes
- 4 teaspoons instant coffee granules
- 2 tablespoons hemp seeds

Method:

1. Add banana, milk, pumpkin pie spice, pumpkin, maple syrup, ice, coffee and hemp seeds into a blender.
2. Blend for 30-40 seconds or until smooth.
3. Pour into tall glasses and serve.

13. Raspberry Anti-Cancer Smoothie

Ingredients:

- 1 carrot, peeled and chopped
- 1 cup fresh raspberries
- 4 tablespoons flaxseed oil
- ½ cup protein powder of your choice
- 1 cup lukewarm filtered water
- 1 cup yogurt or kefir
- 2 teaspoons vitamin C crystals
- 6 small slices fresh beetroots
- 4 thin slices ginger
- 2 tablespoons sweetener of your choice (optional)

Method:

1. Add the carrot, raspberries, flaxseed oil, protein powder, water, yogurt, vitamin C crystals, beetroots, ginger and sweetener (if using) into the blender.
2. Blend for 30-40 seconds or until smooth.
3. Pour into tall glasses and serve.

14. Very Berry Antioxidant Smoothie

Ingredients:

- 2 cups frozen raspberries
- 7-8 strawberries
- ½ cup frozen cherries, pitted or use extra raspberries
- 4 teaspoons fresh ginger, grated
- 1 ½ cups almond milk, unsweetened or rice milk
- 2 teaspoons ground flaxseeds
- 3 tablespoons honey
- 1 ½ tablespoons lemon juice

Method:

1. Add raspberries, strawberries, cherries, ginger, milk, ground flaxseeds, honey and lemon juice into a blender.
2. Blend for 30-40 seconds or until smooth.
3. Pour into tall glasses and serve immediately.

15. Berry Overload Smoothie

Ingredients:

- 1 ½ cups almond milk or skim milk
- ½ cup raspberries, fresh or frozen
- ½ cup blueberries, fresh or frozen
- ½ cup blackberries, fresh or frozen
- 5-6 strawberries, fresh or frozen
- 2 tablespoons chia seeds
- 2 scoops whey protein powder (optional)
- Ice cubes as required
- 2 teaspoons honey
- ½ cup orange juice

Method:

1. Add milk, raspberries, blueberries, blackberries, strawberries, chia seeds, protein powder, ice cubes, honey and orange juice into a blender.
2. Blend for 30-40 seconds or until smooth.
3. Pour into tall glasses and serve immediately.

16. Vegetable Blast

Ingredients:

- 1 medium carrot, peeled and chopped
- 1 small red onion, peeled and chopped
- 2 apples, chopped
- 2 cups spinach or kale or any other dark leafy greens of your choice, chopped
- ½ cup cilantro, chopped
- 2 stalks celery, chopped
- 1 jalapeño pepper, chopped
- 2 cloves garlic, peeled
- 2-3 inches fresh turmeric peeled and sliced) or ½ teaspoon ground turmeric powder
- 1 red bell pepper, chopped
- 4 tomatoes, chopped
- Zest of 1 lime, grated
- 2 cups water
- 1 cup ice cubes or as required

Method:

1. Add spinach, carrot, apple garlic, celery, onion, cilantro, water, jalapeño pepper, turmeric, bell pepper, tomatoes and lime zest into a blender.
2. Blend for 30-40 seconds or until smooth. Add more water to make it thinner if you desire.
3. Pour into tall glasses and serve with crushed ice.

17. Fruit and Vegetable Smoothie

Ingredients:

- ½ cup celery, chopped
- 1 cup carrots, chopped
- 4 large tomatoes, chopped
- 1 teaspoon hot sauce
- ½ cup apple juice
- 1 cup tomato juice

Method:

1. Add celery, carrots and tomatoes into the blender.
2. Add hot sauce, apple juice and tomato juice into the blender.
3. Blend for 30-40 seconds until smooth.
4. Pour into tall glasses and serve with crushed ice.

18. Red Smoothie

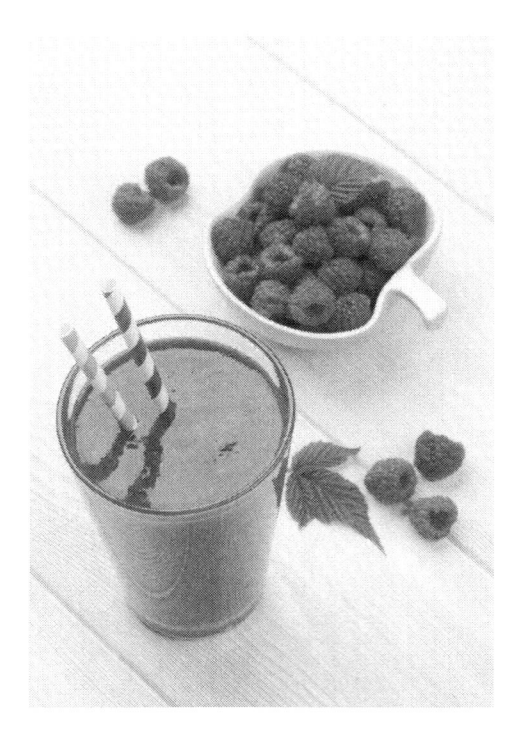

Ingredients:

- 1 small beetroot, peeled and chopped
- 1 small avocado, peeled and chopped
- 2 handfuls goji berries
- 1 cup raspberries
- 20 red grapes, seedless
- 4 small broccoli florets
- 1 ½ cups coconut water
- 2 teaspoon olive oil

Method:

1. Add goji berries, raspberries, avocado, beetroot, red grapes, broccoli, coconut water and oil into a blender.
2. Blend for 30-40 seconds or until smooth. Add more coconut water if required, to thin the smoothie.
3. Pour into tall glasses and serve with crushed ice.

19. Roasted Vegetable Smoothie

Ingredients:

- 1 small zucchini or summer squash, chopped, 1-inch pieces
- 2 medium carrots, chopped, 1-inch pieces
- ½ bunch celery, chopped, 1-inch pieces
- 2 red bell pepper, chopped, 1-inch pieces
- 1 jalapeño pepper or Serrano pepper (optional), chopped
- 1 large tomato, quartered
- 1 can diced tomatoes with its juice, unsalted
- ½ cup fresh cilantro
- 2 tablespoons lime juice
- ¼ cup water or more if required

Method:

1. Spread zucchini, carrot, celery, bell pepper, jalapeño pepper and tomatoes on a baking sheet.
2. Roast in a preheated oven at 425 F for about 25-30 minutes or until done. Shake the vegetables half way through roasting.
3. Remove the baking sheet from the oven and cool completely.
4. Transfer into a blender.
5. Add canned tomatoes, cilantro, lime juice and water.

6. Blend for 30-40 seconds or until smooth. Add more water if required if you like a smoothie of thinner consistency.
7. Pour into tall glasses and serve with crushed ice.

20. Spicy Anti-Inflammatory Smoothie

Ingredients:

- 1 medium avocado, peeled and chopped
- 1 cup fresh or frozen cherries, pitted
- 1 inch piece ginger, peel and slice
- 1 cup fresh or frozen blueberries
- 1 cup fresh or frozen papaya chunks
- 2 tablespoon chia seeds
- 1 teaspoon turmeric powder
- ½ teaspoon cayenne pepper
- 2 cups green tea, chilled
- 1 teaspoon cinnamon powder
- A dash of salt
- 2 teaspoons honey
- 2 cups baby spinach
- 1 tablespoon coconut oil

Method:

1. Add avocado, cherries, ginger, blueberries, papaya, avocado, ginger, chia seeds, turmeric powder, cayenne pepper, green tea, cinnamon, salt, honey, cherries, spinach and coconut oil into a blender.
2. Blend for 30-40 seconds or until smooth. Add more water if required if you like a smoothie of thinner consistency.
3. Pour into tall glasses and serve with crushed ice.

21. Grapefruit Berry Mint

Ingredients:

- 1 medium grapefruit, peeled, deseeded and quartered
- 2 cups frozen strawberries
- 1 cup coconut milk
- ¼ cup fresh mint leaves

Method:

1. Add grapefruit, strawberries, coconut milk and mint leaves into a blender.
2. Blend for 30-40 seconds or until smooth.
3. Add more coconut milk if required if you like a smoothie of thinner consistency.
4. Pour into tall glasses and serve with crushed ice.

22. Papaya Guava Smoothie

Ingredients:

- 2 inch piece ginger, peeled and sliced
- 2 sprigs parsley, chopped
- 2 large guavas, chopped
- 1 teaspoon lemon juice
- 2 teaspoons pure maple syrup or brown sugar or stevia
- 2 cups ripe papaya chunks
- 2 teaspoons flaxseeds

Method:

1. Add the ginger, parsley, guavas, lemon juice, maple syrup, papaya chunks and flaxseeds into a blender.
2. Blend for 30-40 seconds until smooth.
3. Pour into tall glasses and serve with crushed ice.

23. Loaded Anti-oxidant Smoothie

Ingredients:

- 4 cups ripe pineapple chunks
- 6 inches fresh ginger root (peeled and sliced) or 4 teaspoons ginger powder
- 6 inches fresh turmeric root (peeled and sliced) or 4 teaspoons turmeric powder
- 2 cups freshly squeezed orange juice
- 1 teaspoon pepper powder
- 2 teaspoons coconut oil, melted

Method:

1. Add pineapple, ginger, turmeric, orange juice, pepper powder and coconut oil into a blender.
2. Blend for 30-40 seconds or until smooth.
3. Add some water if required if you like a smoothie of thinner consistency.
4. Pour into tall glasses and serve with crushed ice.

24. Watermelon Smoothie

Ingredients:

- 3 cups water melon chunks, frozen
- 2-3 tablespoons lemon juice
- A pinch salt (optional)
- 2 cups coconut water
- A handful mint leaves

Method:

1. Add watermelon, lemon juice, salt and coconut water into the blender.
2. Blend for 30-40 seconds or until smooth.
3. Add mint leaves and pulse for 4-5 seconds.
4. Pour into tall glasses. Serve with crushed ice.

25. Pumpkin Smoothie

Ingredients:

- 2 frozen bananas, peeled and sliced
- 1 cup yogurt
- 1 cup pumpkin puree
- 2 cups milk
- 2 tablespoons maple syrup
- ½ teaspoon vanilla extract
- ½ teaspoon pumpkin pie spice or cinnamon

Method:

1. Add yogurt, pumpkin puree, milk, maple syrup, vanilla, pumpkin pie spice and bananas into a blender.
2. Blend for 30-40 seconds or until smooth.
3. Pour into tall glasses and serve immediately.

26. Sweet Potato Smoothie

Ingredients:

- 2 ripe bananas, peeled and sliced
- 2 cups roasted sweet potato, chunks or pureed
- 2 cups milk of your choice
- ¼ teaspoon ground cinnamon
- 1 teaspoon vanilla extract
- Ice cubes, as required

Method:

1. Add the bananas, potato chunks, milk, cinnamon, vanilla extract and ice cubes into a blender.
2. Blend for 30-40 seconds or until smooth.
3. Pour into tall glasses and serve immediately.

27. Strawberry Apple Smoothie

Ingredients:

- 2 zucchini, chopped into small pieces
- 2 red apples, cored and sliced
- 6 ounces strawberries
- 2 teaspoons maqui berry powder
- 2 cups ice
- Juice of a lime
- 2 cups water

Method:

1. Add zucchini, strawberries, maqui berry powder, ice, apples, lime juice and water into a blender.
2. Blend for 30-40 seconds or until smooth.
3. Pour into tall glasses and serve immediately with crushed ice.

28. Garlic Veggie Smoothie

Ingredients:

- 4 cloves garlic, peeled
- 1 avocado, chopped
- 2 medium cucumbers, chopped
- 1 large apple, chopped
- ½ cup mint leaves

Method:

1. Add garlic, cucumber, avocado, apple and mint into the blender.
2. Blend for 30-40 seconds or until smooth.
3. Pour into tall glasses and serve immediately with crushed ice.

29. Berry Flaxseed and Pomegranate Smoothie

Ingredients:

- 6 strawberries, chopped
- 1 small avocado, peeled and chopped
- ½ cup cold green tea
- ½ cup blueberries, fresh or frozen
- 4 teaspoons shelled hemp seeds
- 2 tablespoons goji berries
- ½ teaspoon gingko powder (optional)
- 2 teaspoons acai berry powder
- 1 teaspoon coconut oil
- 1 teaspoon flaxseed oil
- ½ cup pomegranate juice

Method:

30. Add strawberries, avocado, green tea, blueberries, hemp seed, goji berries, gingko (optional) acai, oils and pomegranate juice into the blender.
31. Blend for 30-40 seconds until smooth.
32. Pour into tall glasses and serve with crushed ice.

30. Rosemary Green Smoothie

Ingredients:

- 2 medium bananas, peeled and sliced
- 2 sprigs fresh rosemary, chopped
- 2 cups water
- 2 cups frozen blueberries
- 1 cup frozen mango chunks
- Honey or maple syrup or stevia to taste (optional)
- A pinch salt
- 2 tablespoons flaxseeds or chia seeds
- 2 scoops green super food powder (optional)
- 2 teaspoons coconut oil

Method:

1. Add bananas, water, blueberries, mango, rosemary, sweetener, salt, flaxseeds, green super food powder and coconut oil into a blender.
2. Blend for 30-40 seconds or until smooth.
3. Pour into tall glasses and serve immediately

31. Spicy Tomato Smoothie

Ingredients:

- 1 cup tomatoes, chopped
- 1 small cucumber, chopped
- 1 avocado, chopped
- 2/3 cup spinach, chopped
- Juice of a lemon
- 2 teaspoons hot sauce

Method:

1. Add tomatoes, cucumber, avocado, spinach and lemon juice into a blender.
2. Blend for 30-40 seconds or until smooth.
3. Pour into tall glasses and serve with crushed ice.

32. Veggie Smoothie

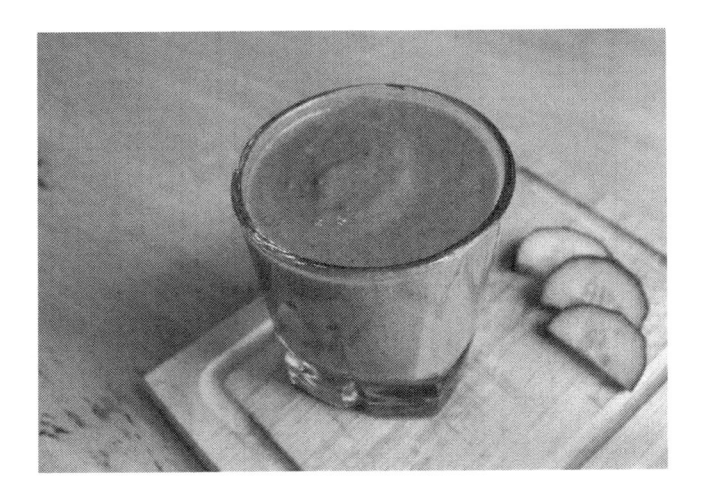

Ingredients:

- 2 carrots, peeled and chopped
- 1 small beetroot, chopped
- 2 cucumbers, chopped
- 2 tomatoes, chopped
- 1 cup spinach, chopped
- 2 cups kombucha or kefir water or raw apple juice or water

Method:

1. Add carrots, beetroot, cucumbers, tomatoes and spinach into the blender. Add raw apple juice or kefir water to the mix and blend for 30-40 seconds or until smooth.
2. Pour into tall glasses and serve with crushed ice.

33. Anti-inflammatory Green Smoothie

Ingredients:

- ½ avocado, peeled and chopped
- 6 cups spinach
- ½ pineapple
- 2 tablespoons chia seeds
- 4 inches fresh turmeric or 2 teaspoons turmeric powder
- ½ cup fresh cilantro
- 3-4 inches fresh ginger
- ½ teaspoon freshly ground pepper

Method:

1. Add avocado, spinach, pineapple, chia seeds, turmeric, cilantro, ginger and pepper into the blender.
2. Blend for 30-40 seconds or until smooth.
3. Pour into tall glasses and serve immediately.

34. Pumpkin Cranberry Smoothie

Ingredients:

- 2 apples, chopped
- 1 orange, peeled and segmented (save pith)
- ½ cup cashews
- 2 cups nondairy milk of your choice
- ½ cup frozen fresh cranberries
- 4 tablespoons coconut cream or coconut butter
- Stevia to taste
- 1 ½ teaspoons ground cinnamon

Method:

1. Soak cashews in bowl of water for 2-3 hours. Drain the water and add into a blender.
2. Add remaining ingredients into the blender.
3. Blend for 30-40 seconds or until smooth. Add some more milk if you like a smoothie of thinner consistency.
4. Pour into tall glasses and serve with crushed ice.

35. Apple and Spinach Smoothie

Ingredients:

- 2 apples, chopped
- 2 cups egg whites, pasteurized
- 4 cups baby spinach
- 2 tablespoons peanut butter
- 2 tablespoons pureed avocado
- Ice cubes, as required

Method:

1. Add egg whites, apples, spinach, peanut butter, avocado and ice cubes into a blender.
2. Blend for 30-40 seconds or until smooth.
3. Pour into tall glasses and serve immediately.

36. Cancer Killer Smoothie

Ingredients:

- 1 cup watermelon, chopped
- 1 cup beet, chopped
- 2 cups fresh pineapple pieces, chopped
- 2 cups baby spinach
- 20 blueberries
- 8 strawberries
- 20 goji berries
- 1 cup beets
- 4 tablespoons hemp powder
- ½ cup watermelon juice
- 2 tablespoons black chia seeds
- 1/3 cup almonds

Method:

1. Add watermelon, beet and pineapple and into a blender and blend for 30 seconds.
2. Add spinach, the berries, hemp powder, chia seed and almonds and blend for another minute or until it becomes smooth.
3. Pour into tall glasses and serve immediately.

37. Fruit Salad Smoothie

Ingredients:

- 4 pears, chilled and chopped
- 4 apples, chilled and chopped
- 1 avocado, peeled and chopped
- 1 stalk celery
- ½ cup cucumber pieces
- 2 cups baby spinach
- 2 small bunches watercress
- 8 ice cubes

Method:

1. Add pears, apples, avocado, celery, cucumber, spinach, watercress and ice cubes to a blender
2. Blend for 30-40 seconds or until smooth.
3. Pour into tall glasses and serve immediately.

38. Cooling Watermelon Smoothie

Ingredients:

- pounds ripe watermelon, chopped
- medium cucumbers, peeled and chopped
- 1 cup celery leaves
- ½ cup fresh mint leaves, chopped finely
- tablespoons lemon juice
- 2 tablespoons flaxseeds, crushed

Method:

1. Add watermelon, cucumber and celery into a blender.
2. Blend for 30-40 seconds or until smooth.
3. Pour into tall glasses.
4. Add mint leaves into the glasses. Stir well.
5. Sprinkle flaxseeds and serve immediately.

39. Immune Boosting Graviola Super Smoothie

Ingredients:

- 3 green apples, chopped
- 1 avocado, chopped
- 4 cups spinach or kale
- 3 cups coconut water or fresh apple juice
- 2 teaspoons Graviola powder

Method:

1. Add apples, avocado, spinach, water and Graviola powder into a blender.
2. Blend for 30-40 seconds or until smooth.
3. Pour into tall glasses.

40. Maca Smoothie

Ingredients:

- 1 avocado or mango, peeled and chopped
- 1 cup spinach leaves, torn
- 2 dozen strawberries, halved or quartered
- 1 cup almonds
- teaspoons organic Raw maca powder
- tablespoons plain yogurt

Method:

1. Add avocado, almonds, strawberries, maca powder, spinach and yogurt into a blender.
2. Blend for 30-40 seconds or until smooth.
3. Pour into tall glasses.
4. Serve with crushed ice.

41. Super Smoothie

Ingredients:

- dates, pitted
- 2 bananas, peeled and sliced
- 2 cups kale leaves, torn
- 2 cups spinach, torn
- 2 cups frozen blueberries
- 2/3 cup water or coconut water or almond milk
- 2 teaspoons spirulina

Method:

1. Add banana, blueberries, spinach, kale, coconut water/milk that you are using and spirulina into a blender.
2. Blend for 30-40 seconds or until smooth.
3. Pour into tall glasses.
4. Serve with crushed ice.

42. Chai Blackberry Smoothie

Ingredients:

- 1 banana, peeled and sliced
- 2 cups fresh blackberries
- 2 tablespoons chia seeds + extra to garnish
- Ice cubes, as required
- 2/3 cup plain yogurt
- A little milk (optional)

Method:

1. Add banana, blackberries, chia seeds, ice cubes, yogurt and milk into a blender.
2. Blend for 30-40 seconds or until smooth.
3. Pour into tall glasses.
4. Serve with crushed ice.

Chapter 3: Anti-Cancer Smoothie Bowl Recipes

1. Butternut Squash, Carrot and Turmeric Smoothie Bowl

Ingredients:

- 1 cup finely grated carrot or frozen diced carrots
- 1 cup frozen mango chunks
- 2 cups frozen diced butternut squash
- 1 ½ cups almond milk or light coconut milk or water
- 4 teaspoons ground turmeric
- ½ teaspoon sea salt
- ¼ teaspoon pepper powder
- 2 scoops vanilla protein powder
- 2 inches fresh ginger, peeled, sliced
- 1 teaspoon ground cinnamon (optional)

Toppings (optional): Use any

- 2 tablespoons granola
- 2 tablespoons almond butter
- A handful almonds, chopped
- 2 tablespoons hemp seeds
- 3-4 dates, pitted, chopped
- Mulberries etc.

Method:

1. Add carrots, mango, butternut squash, almond milk, turmeric powder, salt, pepper, protein powder, ginger and cinnamon into a blender.
2. Blend for 30-40 seconds or until smooth.
3. Pour into 2 bowls.
4. Top with optional toppings and serve with a spoon.

2. Enlighten Smoothie Bowl

Ingredients:

For smoothie:

- 1 large frozen banana, peeled and sliced
- 3 cups, fresh or frozen mixed berries or mixed fruit of your choice
- 6 tablespoons coconut milk or almond milk + extra if required
- 2 scoops plant based protein powder or 4 tablespoons almond or natural peanut butter (optional)
- 3-4 ice cubes (optional)

Optional toppings: Use at least 2 of these

- 2 tablespoons chia seeds
- 2 tablespoons shredded coconut, unsweetened
- 2 tablespoons hemp seeds
- 4 tablespoons granola
- 2-4 tablespoons nut or seed butter
- Banana slices
- Berries of your choice
- Nuts of your choice etc.

Method:

1. Add berries and banana into a blender. Blend for 30-40 seconds until smooth.
2. Add milk, protein powder and ice cubes if using and blend until smooth.
3. Divide into 2 serving bowls.
4. Top with the toppings of your choice and serve.

3. Black Forest Smoothie Bowl

Ingredients:

- 1 frozen banana, peeled, sliced
- 1 cup frozen cherries
- ½ cup black cherry yogurt or vanilla yogurt
- 1 cup almond milk, unsweetened
- 2 scoops chocolate protein powder
- 2 tablespoons almond butter
- 2 tablespoons chia seeds
- 2 tablespoons cocoa powder
- Ice cubes, as required (optional)

Optional toppings: Use at least 2 of these

- 2 tablespoons chia seeds
- 1 tablespoon cacao nibs
- 2 tablespoons hemp seeds
- 4 tablespoons granola
- 2-4 tablespoons nut or seed butter
- Banana slices
- Cherries
- Nuts of your choice etc.

Method:

1. Add cherries and banana into a blender. Blend for 30-40 seconds until smooth.

2. Add milk, protein powder, almond butter, chia seeds, cocoa powder and ice cubes if using and blend until smooth.
3. Divide into 2 serving bowls.
4. Top with optional toppings of your choice and serve.

4. Tropical Smoothie Bowl

Ingredients:

- 1 cup frozen pineapple
- 1 cup frozen papaya
- 1 ½ cups frozen mango
- 2 ½ cups fresh orange juice
- 2 tablespoons Lucama powder (optional)
- ½ teaspoon ground turmeric
- ¼ cup hemp seeds

For topping: Use at least 2 of these

- A few slices fresh mango
- A few slices fresh pineapple
- ¼ cup mixed seeds of your choice
- ¼ cup cashew nuts
- Fresh melon balls

Method:

1. Add pineapple, papaya, mango, orange juice, Lucama powder, turmeric and hemp seeds into a blender.
2. Blend for 30-40 seconds until smooth.
3. Divide the smoothie into 2 bowls. Chill until use.
4. Place the toppings on top.
5. Serve.

5. Chocolate Hazelnut Hemp Smoothie Bowl

Ingredients:

For smoothie:

- 4 bananas, sliced, frozen
- 4 tablespoons hemp protein
- 1 ½ cups almond milk
- ½ cup hazelnuts, soaked in water for 30 minutes
- 4 tablespoons raw cacao powder
- 7-8 large medjool dates, pitted, soaked in water for 15 minutes

For topping:

- ¼ cup hazelnuts, chopped
- 2 small bananas
- 2 tablespoons hemp seeds
- 2 tablespoons cacao nibs

Method:

1. Add hemp protein, banana, milk, nuts, cacao and dates into a blender.
2. Blend for 30-40 seconds until smooth.
3. Divide and pour into 2 bowls. Place the toppings as per taste.
4. Serve.

6. Raspberry Almond Butter Smoothie Bowl

Ingredients:

- 2 large bananas, peeled and sliced
- 10 strawberries, sliced
- 3 cups raspberries
- 1 cup soy milk
- 2 tablespoons honey + extra to drizzle
- 4 tablespoons almond butter
- ¼ cup shredded coconut
- 1 cup ice cubes
- ½ cup granola

Method:

1. Add banana, 2 cups raspberries, soymilk, honey, almond butter and ice into a blender.
2. Blend for 30-40 seconds or until smooth.
3. Divide into 2 bowls.
4. Sprinkle coconut, granola and remaining raspberries on top. Place strawberry slices on top.
5. Top with honey and serve.

7. Cream n Strawberry Smoothie Bowl

Ingredients:

- 2 cups strawberries (frozen)
- 1 cup yogurt
- ½ cup milk
- ½ teaspoon pure vanilla extract
- 2 tablespoons maple syrup + extra to drizzle
- 1 cup cornflakes
- 2 teaspoons chia seeds
- 2 tablespoons pumpkin seeds
- ¼ cup almonds
- 10 strawberries, sliced + extra to top
- ½ cup blueberries

Method:

1. Add strawberries, yogurt, milk, vanilla and maple syrup into a blender.
2. Blend for 30-40 seconds or until smooth.
3. Divide into 2 bowls.
4. Sprinkle cornflakes, chia seeds, pumpkin seeds and almonds on top.
5. Place strawberry slices and blueberries on top.
6. Drizzle some more maple syrup and yogurt if desired.
7. Serve.

8. Red Berry Smoothie Bowl

Ingredients:

For smoothie:

- 2 cups water
- 4 rooibos tea bags
- 1 cup goji berries
- 1 cup frozen raspberries
- 2 cups frozen strawberries
- 12 ounces coconut milk yogurt
- 6 tablespoons hemp seeds

For topping:

- Few slices fresh strawberries
- A large handful raspberries
- Any other toppings of your choice

Method:

1. Boil the water and turn off the heat. Drop the tea bags in it. Cover and set aside for 10 minutes to steep.
2. Discard the tea bags. Transfer into a bowl.
3. Add goji berries and stir. Cover and place in the refrigerator overnight.
4. Add all the berries, chilled tea, yogurt and hemp seeds into a blender.
5. Blend for 30-40 seconds or until smooth.

6. Divide the smoothie into 3-4 bowls.
7. Garnish with strawberries and raspberries.
8. Top with toppings of your choice and serve.

9. Kale and Avocado Smoothie Bowl

Ingredients:

- 2 bananas, peeled and sliced
- 1 avocado, peeled and chopped
- 2 kiwis, peeled and sliced
- 2 cups kale leaves, discard hard stems and ribs
- 2 tablespoons agave nectar + extra to drizzle
- 2 cups almond milk
- 1 cup ice cubes
- 2 teaspoons chia seeds
- 1 cup raspberries

Method:

1. Add kale, 1 banana, agave, almond milk, ice and avocado into a blender.
2. Blend for 30-40 seconds or until smooth.
3. Divide the smoothie into 2 bowls.
4. Garnish with kiwi slices, 1 banana, chia seeds and raspberries.
5. Drizzle agave on top and serve.

10. Pineapple, Peach and Banana Smoothie Bowl

Ingredients:

- 2 bananas, peeled and sliced
- 1 peach, sliced
- 2 cups pineapple chunks (frozen)
- 2 tablespoons honey + extra to drizzle
- ½ cup coconut water
- ¼ cup sunflower seeds
- ½ rice cereal (rice Krispies will do)
- 1 cup blackberries

Method:

1. Add banana, peach, pineapple, honey and coconut water into a blender.
2. Blend for 30-40 seconds or until smooth.
3. Divide the smoothie into 2 bowls.
4. Garnish with peach slices, sunflower seeds, rice cereal and blackberries.
5. Drizzle some honey on top and serve.

11. Dark Cherry Smoothie Bowl

Ingredients:

For smoothie:

- 4 cups frozen cherries
- 1 ½ cups coconut water
- 2 bananas, peeled and sliced

For toppings:

- 16 whole cherries
- ½ cup almond slices
- ½ cup coconut flakes
- ½ cup raw cacao nibs

Method:

1. To make smoothie: Pit the cherries.
2. Add cherries, bananas and coconut water into a blender.
3. Blend for 30-40 seconds or until smooth.
4. Divide the smoothie into 2 bowls.
5. Sprinkle the toppings on top.
6. Serve.

12. Mixed Berry Smoothie Bowl

Ingredients:

- 3 cups frozen mixed berries
- ½ cup plain yogurt + extra to drizzle
- ½ cup pomegranate juice
- 1 peach, sliced
- ¼ cup pumpkin seeds
- ¼ cup dried mulberries
- 1 cup blueberries

Method:

1. Add berries, yogurt and pomegranate juice into a blender.
2. Blend for 30-40 seconds or until smooth.
3. Divide the smoothie into 2 bowls.
4. Garnish with peach slices, pumpkin seeds, mulberries and blueberries.
5. Drizzle some yogurt on top and serve.

13. Green Smoothie Bowl

Ingredients:

- 1-½ cups assorted kale like curly and lacinato etc, torn
- ½ ripe avocado, chopped
- ½ cup coconut milk or coconut water or unsweetened almond milk
- ½ cup spinach
- ½ small banana, frozen
- 1 Brazil nut
- ½ teaspoon ground cinnamon
- ¼ teaspoon ground ginger
- 2 medjool dates, pitted
- 1 teaspoon moringa powder
- A pinch salt
- ½ scoop protein powder or collagen powder
- 2 teaspoons almond butter
- ½ teaspoon turmeric powder
- Ice cubes as required
- Kiwi slices to serve
- 1 teaspoon chia seeds to serve
- 1 teaspoon coconut flakes, unsweetened to serve
- Sweetener of your choice (optional)

Method:

1. Add all the ingredients except kiwi, chia seeds and coconut flakes into a blender.
2. Blend for 30-40 seconds or until smooth.
3. Pour into a bowl. Sprinkle chia seeds and coconut flakes. Top with kiwi slices and serve.

14. Peach, Orange, and Berry Smoothie Bowl

Ingredients:

- 3 cups frozen peach
- 1 cup orange juice
- 2 bananas, peeled, sliced
- 1 cup blueberries
- 1 cup blackberries
- 4 tablespoons hemp seeds
- ½ cup walnuts
- Honey to drizzle

Method:

1. Add peach, orange juice and banana into a blender.
2. Blend for 30-40 seconds or until smooth.
3. Pour into 2 bowls.
4. Scatter berries, hemp seeds and walnuts.
5. Drizzle some honey on top and serve.

15. Super Food Avocado Smoothie Bowl with Cashew Cream

Ingredients:

For cashew cream:

- ¼ cup cashews + extra to top, toasted
- 3 tablespoons light coconut milk

For smoothie bowl:

- 2 tablespoons mashed avocado
- 6 tablespoons vanilla almond milk
- 2 tablespoons 2% vanilla Greek yogurt
- 1 tablespoon vanilla protein powder
- 2 kale leaves, discard hard ribs and stem, torn
- ¼ small banana, sliced, frozen
- A pinch salt

For topping:

- Pomegranate seeds
- Coconut flakes

Method:

1. Place cashews in a bowl and pour water over it. Cover the bowl and refrigerate overnight. Drain and add into a small blender.
2. Add coconut milk and salt into a large blender and blend until smooth and creamy.
3. Add rest of the ingredients into the larger blender and blend until smooth and creamy.
4. Pour into a bowl. Add about 2 tablespoons of cashew cream and swirl lightly with a blunt knife.
5. Sprinkle the extra cashew, coconut flakes and pomegranate seeds on top and serve with any other toppings of your choice if desired.

16. Pitaya Breakfast Bowl

Ingredients:

For smoothie:

- 3 bananas, peeled and sliced
- 4 packages frozen Pitaya puree (Dragon fruit)
- 1 cup frozen berries or your choice
- 4 tablespoons hemp seed powder or nut butter of your choice
- 1 cup almond milk

For topping:

- A few banana slices
- ½ cup fresh or frozen berries, thawed

Method:

1. Add all the ingredients into a blender.
2. Blend for 30-40 seconds or until smooth.
3. Divide the smoothie into 4 bowls. Chill if desired.
4. Top with banana slices and berries.
5. You can also sprinkle any other toppings of your choice.

17. Peach-Raspberry Smoothie Bowl

Ingredients:

- 1 cup frozen peach slices
- 4 cups frozen raspberries
- 1 cup plain whole milk yogurt
- 2 tablespoons raw honey
- 1 medium zucchini, chopped
- 2 tablespoons ground flaxseeds
- ¼ teaspoon salt
- 2 teaspoons vanilla extract

Method:

1. Add peach, raspberries, yogurt, honey, zucchini, flaxseeds, salt and vanilla into a blender.
2. Blend for 30-40 seconds or until smooth.
3. Divide into 4 bowls.
4. Sprinkle toppings of your choice and serve.

Chapter 4: Anti-Cancer Layered Smoothie Recipes

1. 2 layered Mango – Peach and Strawberry – Banana Smoothie

Ingredients:

For mango peach layer:

- 4 very ripe mangoes, peeled and chopped
- 4 very ripe peaches, peeled and chopped
- 2 cups mango or peach nectar, peeled and chopped
- Lime juice to taste
- 2 cups 2% Greek yogurt
- Honey to taste

For strawberry banana layer:

- 4 pints strawberries, chopped
- 4 ripe bananas, peeled and sliced
- Lemon juice to taste
- Finely chopped mango, peach and strawberries to garnish

Method:

1. Layer peaches and mangos and all the remaining ingredients for that layer into a blender.
2. Blend for 30-40 seconds or until smooth.

3. Divide and pour into tall glasses.
4. Clean the blender..
5. Add strawberries, banana and lime juice into a blender and blend until smooth.
6. Pour into the glasses over the mango peach layer.
7. Garnish with finely chopped mango, peach and strawberries and serve.

2. Tropical Layered Smoothie

Ingredients:

For blueberry layer:

- 1 cup frozen mango chunks
- 4 tablespoons agave nectar
- 1 cup frozen blueberries
- 1 cup Greek yogurt (law fat)
- 2 tablespoons fresh lime juice

For mango layer:

- 4 tablespoons agave nectar
- 1 cup frozen mango
- 1 cup Greek yogurt
- 2 small bananas, peeled, sliced
- 2 tablespoons fresh lemon juice

For strawberry layer:

- 2 cups frozen strawberries
- 1 cup plain Greek yogurt
- 2 small bananas, peeled, sliced
- 2 tablespoons fresh lemon juice
- 4 tablespoons agave nectar

For toppings: Optional

- A handful blueberries
- A handful pomegranate arils

- 2-3 strawberries, chopped
- A handful finely chopped mangoes

Method:

1. For blueberry layer: Add all the ingredients of blueberry layer into a blender. Blend for 30-40 seconds until smooth and thick.
2. Divide the smoothie equally and pour into 4 glasses. Place the glasses in the freezer. Clean the blender.
3. For mango layer: Add all the ingredients of mango layer into a blender. Blend for 30-40 seconds until smooth and thick.
4. Divide the smoothie equally and pour over the blueberry layer gently. Place the glasses in the freezer. Clean the blender.
5. For strawberry layer: Add all the ingredients of strawberry layer into the blender. Blend for 30-40 seconds or until smooth and thick.
6. Divide the smoothie equally and pour gently over the mango layer. Place the glasses in the freezer.
7. Top with the toppings mentioned above or of your choice and serve.

3. Sunrise Smoothie

Ingredients:

- 3 cups water melon cubes, deseeded
- 2 cups cantaloupe cubes, deseeded
- ½ cup orange juice
- 1 cup low fat plain yogurt
- 4 small wedges of cantaloupe or water melon to serve

Method:

1. Add watermelon cubes into the blender.
2. Blend for 30-40 seconds or until smooth.
3. Divide into tall glass.
4. Clean the blender.
5. Add cantaloupe, orange juice and yogurt into the blender.
6. Gently pour the cantaloupe puree over the watermelon in the glass. Do not stir.
7. Garnish with cantaloupe or watermelon and serve immediately.

4. Super Healthy Rainbow Smoothie

Ingredients:

For blue / purple layer:

- 1 1/3 cups frozen blueberries
- ½ cup cashew milk or almond milk
- 2 tablespoons almond butter

For green layer:

- 1 avocado, peeled, pitted, chopped
- 2 cups fresh baby spinach
- 2 bananas, sliced, frozen

For yellow layer:

- 2 2/3 cups frozen mango
- ½ cup shredded coconut, unsweetened
- 6 tablespoons full fat coconut milk

For red layer:

- 2 cups frozen raspberries
- ½ cup cashew milk or almond milk
- 4 tablespoons hemp hearts

For pink layer:

- 2 cups frozen cherries, pitted
- 1 teaspoon vanilla extract
- 2 cups frozen strawberries
- ½ cup cashew milk

Optional toppings: Use any

- Kiwi slices
- Blueberries
- Cherries
- Strawberry slices
- Coconut whipped cream
- Sprinkles etc.

Method:

1. For blue layer: Add blueberries, milk and almond butter into a blender. Blend for 30-40 seconds or until smooth and thick.
2. Take 4 glasses. Divide the smoothie equally and pour into the glasses. Place the glasses in the freezer. Clean the blender.
3. For yellow layer: Add all the ingredients of yellow layer into a blender. Blend for 30-40 seconds until smooth and thick.
4. Divide the smoothie equally and pour over the pink layer gently. Place the glasses in the freezer. Clean the blender.

5. For green layer: Add all the ingredients of green layer into a blender. Blend for 30-40 seconds until smooth and thick.
6. Divide the smoothie equally and pour over the yellow layer gently. Place the glasses in the freezer. Clean the blender.
7. For red layer: Add all the ingredients of red layer into the blender. Blend for 30-40 seconds or until smooth and thick.
8. Divide the smoothie equally and pour gently over the green layer. Place glasses in the freezer.
9. For pink layer: Add all the ingredients of pink layer into a blender. Blend for 30-40 seconds until smooth and thick.
10. Divide the smoothie equally and pour over the green layer gently. Place the glasses in the freezer for 15-20 minutes.
11. Top with the toppings of your choice and serve.

5. Avocado Strawberry Layered Smoothie

Ingredients:

For strawberry layer:

- 3 cups frozen strawberries
- 1 cup water
- 2 bananas, frozen
- 3 teaspoons lemon juice
- 1 tablespoon honey or to taste

For avocado smoothie:

- 2/3 cup almond milk, unsweetened milk
- 5 tablespoons honey
- Ice cubes, as required
- 3 cups chopped avocado
- 2 tablespoons lemon juice
- 2 teaspoons pure vanilla extract

Method:

1. For strawberry layer: Add all the ingredients of strawberry layer into a blender. Blend for 30-40 seconds or until smooth and thick.
2. Divide the smoothie equally and pour into glasses. Place the glasses in the freezer. Clean the blender.

3. For avocado layer: Add all the ingredients of avocado layer into a blender. Blend for 30-40 seconds or until smooth and thick.
4. Divide the smoothie equally and pour over the strawberry layer gently.
5. Place the glasses in the freezer for 15 minutes and serve.

6. Berry Beet Smoothie

Ingredients:

Strawberry smoothie:

- 2 bananas, peeled, sliced, frozen
- 2 cups frozen strawberries
- 2 cups frozen pineapple chunks
- ½ - 1 cup milk of your choice or orange juice or water
- 1 cup plain or vanilla Greek yogurt

For beet smoothie:

- 2 cans (15 ounces each) whole beets
- 2 bananas, peeled, sliced, frozen
- ½ - 1 cup milk of your choice or orange juice or water
- 4 cups frozen raspberries
- 1 cup plain or vanilla Greek yogurt

To top:

- 4 toothpicks with leftover fruits inserted in it

Method:

1. For strawberry layer: Add all the ingredients of strawberry layer into a blender. Blend for 30-40 seconds or until smooth and thick.
2. Divide the smoothie equally and pour into glasses. Place the glasses in the freezer. Clean the blender.

3. For beet layer: Add all the ingredients of beet layer into a blender. Blend for 30-40 seconds or until smooth and thick.
4. Divide the smoothie equally and pour over the strawberry layer gently.
5. Place the glasses in the freezer for 15 minutes and serve.
6. Place a toothpick with fruits inserted in it, in each glass.

7. Cherry Mango Smoothie

Ingredients:

For cherry layer:

- 1 cup water
- 2 cups frozen sweet cherries, thawed for 10 minutes

For mango layer:

- 1 ½ cups water
- 2 cups frozen mango, thawed for 10 minutes

Method:

1. For cherry layer: Add cherry and water into the blender.
2. Blend for 30-40 seconds or until smooth.
3. Pour into 2 glasses.
4. Clean the blender.
5. For mango layer: Add mango and water into the blender.
6. Blend for 30-40 seconds or until smooth.
7. Pour over the cherry layer.
8. Chill the glasses in the freezer for 15 minutes.
9. Serve.

8. Hawaiian Berry Smoothie

Ingredients:

For Berry layer:

- 8 ounces berry yogurt
- 2 medium bananas, peeled, sliced, frozen
- 3 cups frozen berries of your choice
- 1/3 cup milk or more if required

For Hawaiian layer:

- 1 ½ oranges, peeled, sliced, deseeded
- 1 ½ cups frozen mango
- 3 bananas, peeled, sliced, frozen
- ½ cup fresh orange juice

Method:

1. For berry layer: Add all the ingredients of berry layer into a blender. Blend for 30-40 seconds or until smooth and thick.
2. Divide the smoothie equally and pour into glasses. Place the glasses in the freezer. Clean the blender.
3. For Hawaiian layer: Add all the ingredients of Hawaiian layer into a blender. Blend for 30-40 seconds or until smooth and thick.
4. Divide the smoothie equally and pour over the berry layer gently.
5. Place the glasses in the freezer for 15 minutes and serve.
6. Place a toothpick with fruits inserted in it, in each glass.

9. Layered Mixed Berry Green Power Smoothie

Ingredients:

For berry layer:

- ¾ cup milk
- 1 small banana, peeled, sliced, frozen
- ½ cup raspberries
- ¼ avocado, peeled, chopped
- ½ cup blueberries
- ½ tablespoon vanilla protein powder

For green layer:

- 1 small banana, peeled, sliced, frozen
- 1 small kiwifruit, peeled, chopped
- ¼ avocado, peeled, chopped
- ¾ cup milk
- ½ cup chopped mango
- 1 cup spinach, loosely packed
- ½ tablespoon vanilla protein powder

Method:

1. For berry layer: Add all the ingredients of berry layer into a blender. Blend for 30-40 seconds or until smooth and thick.
2. Divide the smoothie equally and pour into glasses. Place the glasses in the freezer. Clean the blender.

3. For green layer: Add all the ingredients of green layer into a blender. Blend for 30-40 seconds or until smooth and thick.
4. Divide the smoothie equally and pour over the berry layer gently.
5. Place the glasses in the freezer for 15 minutes if desired and serve or serve immediately.

10. Strawberry Mango Smoothie

Ingredients:

For mango layer:

- 1 large mango, peeled, chopped, frozen
- 6 tablespoons water
- 1 ½ cups orange juice

For strawberry layer:

- 1 cup frozen strawberries
- 2 tablespoons honey or sugar (optional)
- 2 cups orange juice

Method:

1. For mango layer: Add all the ingredients of mango layer into a blender. Blend for 30-40 seconds or until smooth and thick.
2. Divide the smoothie equally and pour into glasses. Place the glasses in the freezer. Clean the blender.
3. For strawberry layer: Add all the ingredients of strawberry layer into a blender. Blend for 30-40 seconds or until smooth and thick.
4. Divide the smoothie equally and pour over the mango layer gently.
5. Serve immediately.

11. Berry, Banana and Kale Smoothie

Ingredients:

For banana-almond layer:

- 4 small bananas, peeled, sliced
- ½ cup semi-skimmed milk
- 1 cup crushed ice
- 20 almonds

For kale- date layer:

- 6-8 medjool dates, pitted, chopped
- ½ cup crushed ice
- 3 cups kale, discard hard stem and ribs, torn

For blueberry layer:

- 1 ½ cups blueberry
- ½ cup crushed ice
- 1/3 cup water

For strawberry layer:

- 2 cups strawberries, hulled
- ½ cup crushed ice
- ½ cup semi-skimmed milk

Method:

1. For banana-almond layer: Add all the ingredients of banana-almond layer into a blender. Blend for 30-40 seconds or until smooth and thick.
2. Divide the smoothie equally and pour into glasses. Place the glasses in the freezer. Clean the blender.
3. For kale-date layer: Add all the ingredients of kale-date layer into a blender. Blend for 30-40 seconds or until smooth and thick.
4. Divide the smoothie equally and pour over the banana-almond layer gently. Clean the blender.
5. For blueberry layer: Add all the ingredients of blueberry layer into a blender. Blend for 30-40 seconds or until smooth and thick.
6. Divide the smoothie equally and pour over the kale-date layer. Place the glasses in the freezer. Clean the blender.
7. For strawberry layer: Add all the ingredients of strawberry layer into a blender. Blend for 30-40 seconds or until smooth and thick.
8. Divide the smoothie equally and pour over the strawberry layer gently.
9. Serve immediately.

12. Multi-layered Smoothie

Ingredients:

For yellow layer:

- 1 cup Greek yogurt
- 3 cups frozen mango

For purple layer:

- 2 bananas, peeled, sliced, frozen
- 1 ½ cups frozen blueberries
- ½ teaspoon vanilla extract
- 1 cup Greek yogurt
- ½ teaspoon cinnamon powder

For pink layer:

- 2 cups frozen raspberries
- Coconut syrup to taste
- 1 cup Greek yogurt

To top: Optional

- Hemp seeds
- Chia seeds
- Cinnamon powder
- Coconut flakes etc.

Method:

1. For yellow layer: Add all the ingredients from the yellow layer into a blender. Blend for 30-40 seconds or until smooth and thick.
2. Divide the smoothie equally and pour into glasses. Place the glasses in the freezer. Clean the blender.
3. For purple layer: Add all the ingredients from the purple layer into a blender. Blend for 30-40 seconds or until smooth and thick.
4. Divide the smoothie equally and pour over the yellow layer. Place the glasses in the freezer. Clean the blender.
5. For pink layer: Add all the ingredients from the pink layer into a blender. Blend for 30-40 seconds or until smooth and thick.
6. Divide the smoothie equally and pour over the purple layer gently.
7. Sprinkle any of optional toppings if desired or any other toppings of your choice.
8. Serve immediately.

13. Chocolate, Banana and Pumpkin Swirl Super Smoothie

Ingredients:

- ½ cup plain Greek yogurt
- 1 banana, peeled, sliced, frozen
- 1 cup milk of your choice
- 2/3 cup pumpkin puree
- Maple syrup to taste
- 1 teaspoon vanilla extract
- ¼ teaspoon ground cinnamon
- 1 teaspoon xanthan gum (optional)
- Ice cubes, as required
- 2 -4 teaspoons cocoa powder + extra to sprinkle

Method:

1. Add yogurt, banana, milk, pumpkin puree, maple syrup, vanilla, cinnamon, xanthan gum and ice cubes into a blender.
2. Blend for 30-40 seconds or until smooth.
3. Pour half the smoothie into a large cup with a spout.
4. Add cocoa powder to the remaining smoothie and blend for a few more seconds until well combined.
5. Make layers of the smoothie, alternating between plain and chocolate smoothie, in 2 glasses.

Chapter 5: Anti-Cancer Dessert Smoothies

1. Roasted Strawberry Smoothie

Ingredients:

- 2 pounds whole strawberries, hulled
- 4 tablespoons sugar
- 4 tablespoons honey
- ½ cup water
- 2 cups whipped cottage cheese
- 2 teaspoons vanilla extract
- 1 large banana, peeled and sliced
- 2 cups ice cubes
- Whipped cream to top (optional)

Method:

1. If the strawberries are very large, cut into 2 halves. Place strawberries in a baking dish. Sprinkle sugar over it and toss well.
2. Roast in a preheated oven at 350 F for about 30 minutes. Turn the strawberries half way through roasting.
3. Remove the dish from the oven and set aside to cool.
4. Add strawberries along with the cooked juice, honey, water, cottage cheese, vanilla, banana and ice cubes into a blender.

5. Blend for 30-40 seconds or until smooth. Add more sweetener if desired while blending.
6. Pour into tall glasses and chill for a while.
7. Serve with whipped cream if desired.

2. Dreamy Strawberry Smoothie Layered with Chia Seed Pudding

Ingredients:

For chia seed pudding:

- 1 ½ cups coconut milk or any other nut milk of your choice
- 2 tablespoons honey
- 6 tablespoons chia seeds

For smoothie:

- 2 cups frozen strawberries
- 2 frozen bananas
- 4 dates, pitted
- ½ cup coconut shreds
- 2/3 cup frozen pomegranate arils
- 1 cup coconut water or water or nut milk of your choice
- 2 teaspoons honey

Method:

1. To make chia seed layer: Divide the milk into 4 bowls (6 tablespoons each).
2. Add 1-½ tablespoons chia seeds into each bowl.
3. Add ½ tablespoon honey into each bowl and stir.
4. Place in the refrigerator for 4-5 hours.
5. To make smoothie layer: Add all the ingredients of smoothie layer into the blender.

6. Blend for 30-40 seconds or until smooth.
7. Divide and pour over the chia pudding layer.
8. Serve.

3. Banana Bread Smoothie

Ingredients:

- 3 bananas, sliced and frozen
- 1 teaspoon ground cinnamon
- ½ cup ice cubes
- 5 tablespoons rolled oats
- 1 teaspoon vanilla extract
- 2 cups almond milk
- 4 tablespoons walnuts, chopped, toasted

Method:

1. Add bananas, cinnamon, ice cubes, rolled oats, vanilla extract and milk into the blender.
2. Blend for 30-40 seconds or until smooth.
3. Pour into tall glasses and serve garnished with walnuts.

4. Kiwi Berry Mousse Smoothie

Ingredients:

<u>For berry layer:</u>

- 2 cups berries of your choice
- 2 teaspoons vanilla extract
- 2 cups coconut water
- 4 tablespoons pure protein powder
- 2 teaspoons acai berry powder

<u>For kiwi mousse layer:</u>

- 6 kiwi fruits
- 1 cup baby spinach leaves
- 2 cups coconut water
- 2 large avocadoes
- 20 mint leaves + extra to garnish

Method:

1. For berry layer: Add all the ingredients of berry layer into a blender. Blend for 30-40 seconds or until smooth and thick.
2. Divide the smoothie equally and pour into glasses. Place the glasses in the freezer. Clean the blender.
3. For kiwi mousse layer: Add all the ingredients of kiwi mousse layer into a blender. Blend for 30-40 seconds or until smooth and thick.

4. Divide the mousse equally and spoon over the berry layer. Garnish with mint leaves.
5. Serve immediately.

5. Apple Pie Smoothie

Ingredients:

- 4 large red apples, sliced
- 2 cups ice cubes
- 1 cup Greek yogurt
- ¼ teaspoon ground nutmeg
- 2 teaspoons ground cinnamon + extra to garnish
- 1/8 teaspoon ground cloves
- ¼ teaspoon ground ginger
- 4 dates, pitted or honey to taste

Method:

1. Add apples, ice, yogurt, all the spices and dates into a blender.
2. Blend for 30-40 seconds or until smooth.
3. Pour into tall glasses and serve sprinkled with cinnamon

6. Fruit Cake Smoothie

Ingredients:

- 1 cup pumpkin puree
- 2 cups coconut or almond milk
- 1 cup blueberry juice
- 1 cup berries of your choice
- 1 banana, peeled, sliced, frozen
- 2 tablespoons chocolate almond or hazelnut butter
- 4 tablespoons cocoa powder
- 4 tablespoons grass fed beef gelatin
- Berries to garnish

Method:

1. Add pumpkin puree, milk and blueberry juice into the blender.
2. Blend for 30-40 seconds until smooth.
3. Add berries, banana, hazelnut butter, cocoa and gelatin and blend again.
4. Pour into tall glasses and garnish with berries. Serve with crushed ice.

7. Pumpkin Pie Smoothie

Ingredients:

- 1 cup pumpkin puree
- 2 bananas, peeled, sliced, frozen
- ½ teaspoon vanilla extract
- ½ teaspoon ground cinnamon + extra to garnish
- Ice cubes, as required
- ½ teaspoon pumpkin pie spice
- 3 cups skim milk, unsweetened
- 4 tablespoons pure maple syrup or honey

Method:

1. Add pumpkin puree, bananas, vanilla, cinnamon, ice cubes, spice, skim milk and honey into the blender.
2. Blend for 30-40 seconds or until smooth. Add more milk if you like a smoothie of thinner consistency.
3. Taste and adjust the spices if necessary.
4. Pour into tall glasses and serve garnished with cinnamon.

8. Peanut Butter and Oatmeal Smoothie

Ingredients:

- 2 large ripe bananas, peeled, sliced
- 4 tablespoons peanut butter
- ½ cup quick cooking oats
- 2 cups plain yogurt
- 1 cup milk
- Honey to taste

Method:

1. Add banana, peanut butter, oats, yogurt, milk and honey into a blender.
2. Blend for 30-40 seconds or until smooth.
3. Pour into tall glasses.
4. Drizzle some more honey on top and serve.

9. Strawberry Cheesecake Smoothie

Ingredients:

- 4 ounces low fat cream cheese
- 1 ½ cups plain fat free Greek yogurt
- 2 tablespoons vanilla extract
- 1 cup low fat milk
- 2 cups frozen strawberries
- 3 tablespoons agave nectar

Method:

1. Add cream cheese, yogurt, milk, strawberries, vanilla extract and agave nectar into a blender.
2. Blend for 30-40 seconds or until smooth.
3. Pour into tall glasses and serve.

10. Brownie Smoothie

Ingredients:

- 2 bananas, peeled, sliced, frozen
- 1 cup cooked black beans
- 2 cups milk of your choice
- 2 tablespoons cocoa powder
- 2 cups frozen cauliflower
- 4 medjool dates, pitted
- 2 tablespoons hemp seeds
- 2 teaspoons ground cinnamon

Method:

1. Add bananas, black beans, milk, cocoa, cauliflower, dates, hemp seeds and cinnamon into a blender.
2. Blend for 30-40 seconds or until smooth.
3. Pour into tall glasses and serve.

11. Super Food Pumpkin Pie Green Smoothie

Ingredients:

- 2 cups pumpkin puree
- 2 tablespoons almond butter
- 2 teaspoons pumpkin pie spice
- ¼ cup pecans, chopped
- 2 teaspoons wheatgrass powder (optional)
- 3 cups almond milk, unsweetened
- 2 cups spinach
- 2 cups ice
- 6 medjool dates, pitted
- 4 tablespoons ground flaxseeds

Method:

1. Add pumpkin puree, almond butter, pumpkin pie spice, pecans, wheatgrass powder, almond milk, spinach, ice, dates and flaxseed powder into a blender.
2. Blend for 30-40 seconds or until smooth.
3. Pour into tall glasses and serve.

12. Chocolate Oatmeal Cookie Smoothie

Ingredients:

- 2 large ripe bananas, peeled, sliced
- 4 tablespoons peanut butter
- ½ cup quick cooking oats
- 2-3 tablespoons cocoa powder, unsweetened
- 2 cups plain yogurt
- 1 cup milk
- Honey to taste

Method:

1. Add banana, peanut butter, oats, cocoa, yogurt, milk and honey into a blender.
2. Blend for 30-40 seconds or until smooth.
3. Pour into tall glasses.
4. Drizzle some more honey on top and serve.

13. Carrot Cake Smoothie

Ingredients:

- 6 medium carrots, peeled, chopped
- 1 banana, peeled, sliced, frozen
- 1 ½ cups milk
- 2 teaspoons honey or maple syrup or 6 pitted dates
- 1 teaspoon ground cinnamon
- ¼ cup walnuts, chopped
- ½ cup nonfat plain Greek yogurt
- ¼ teaspoon ground nutmeg
- Shredded coconut to top

Method:

1. Add carrot, banana, milk, honey, cinnamon, walnuts, yogurt and nutmeg into a blender.
2. Blend for 30-40 seconds or until smooth.
3. Pour into tall glasses.
4. Sprinkle shredded coconut on top and serve.

14. Chocolate Peanut Butter Smoothie

Ingredients:

- 1 cup fat free milk or nondairy milk of your choice
- 3 tablespoons cocoa powder, unsweetened
- 2 medium ripe bananas, peeled, chopped
- 4-6 tablespoons creamy peanut butter, unsalted
- 2 tablespoons honey or agave nectar
- Ice cubes, as required

Method:

1. Add milk, cocoa powder, banana, peanut butter, honey and ice into a blender.
2. Blend for 30-40 seconds or until smooth.
3. Pour into tall glasses and serve.

15. Triple Berry Kefir Smoothie

Ingredients:

- 12 ounces fresh blackberries
- 1 cup pomegranate juice
- 2 cups fresh blueberries
- 20 frozen strawberries
- 2 cups kefir yogurt
- 2 large bananas, peeled, sliced, frozen
- Ice cubes, as required

Method:

1. Add blackberries and pomegranate juice into a blender.
2. Blend for 30-40 seconds or until smooth.
3. Add blueberries, strawberries, kefir, banana and ice and blend until smooth.
4. Pour into glasses and serve.

16. Red Velvet Green Smoothie

Ingredients:

- 2 large beets, peeled, quartered
- 6 tablespoons cocoa powder
- 4 cups spinach
- 2 bananas, peeled, frozen
- 2 cups vanilla almond milk
- 6-8 dates, pitted

Method:

1. Add beets, cocoa powder, spinach, bananas, almond milk and dates into a blender.
2. Blend for 30-40 seconds or until smooth.
3. Pour into tall glasses and serve.

17. Blueberry Cheesecake Smoothie

Ingredients:

- 1 ½ cups frozen blueberries
- 2 cups skim milk
- 1 cup cold water
- 1 cup low fat cottage cheese
- ¼ teaspoon ground cinnamon
- Sweetener of your choice, as required like honey, agave nectar, stevia etc.
- 1 teaspoon vanilla extract

Method:

1. Add blueberries, skim milk, cold water, cottage cheese, cinnamon, sweetener and vanilla into a blender. Blend for 30-40 seconds or until smooth. Add more skim milk if you like a smoothie of thinner consistency.
2. Pour into tall glasses and serve with crushed ice.

Conclusion

I sincerely hope this book was useful and that you will benefit from the anti-cancer diet.

This book gave a brief explanation on cancer nutrients, the importance of including the right nutrients into the diet and a quick overview of guidelines on anti-cancer diets. The chapters concentrate on the numerous healthy homemade anti-cancer smoothies that can help provide you with the required cancer-fighting nutrients.

We also included foods that have anti-cancer properties. The ingredients of the recipes mentioned in the book are cost-effective and are readily available in your kitchen or at the organic farmer's market. Filling your diet with healthy, nutrient packed foods can help you feel better and stronger.

So, what are you waiting for? Try the recipes mentioned in the book and start working towards a nutrient packed diet. The better you eat, the better you will feel!

Finally, if you enjoyed this book then I'd like to ask you for a favor. Will you be kind enough to leave a review for this book on Amazon? It would be greatly appreciated!

Bonus

As a way of saying thanks for your purchase, we're offering a special gift that's exclusive to my readers.

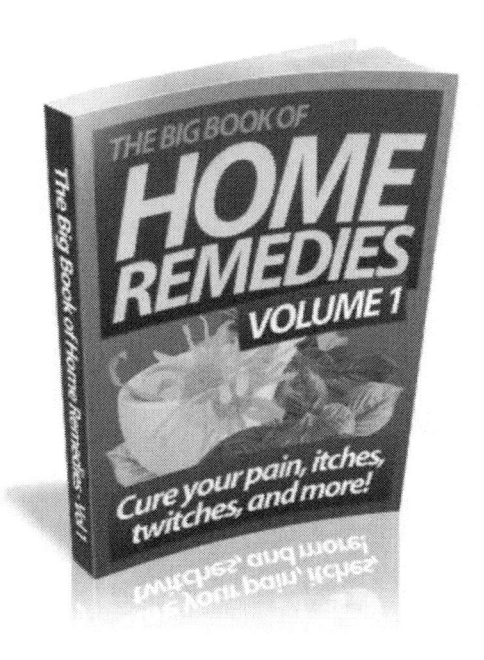

Visit this link below to claim your bonus.

http://dingopublishing.com/heath-freebonus/

Another surprise!

There are free sample chapters of our **favorite** book at the end (from page 140):

Anti-inflammatory Diet for Beginners
by Jonathan Smith

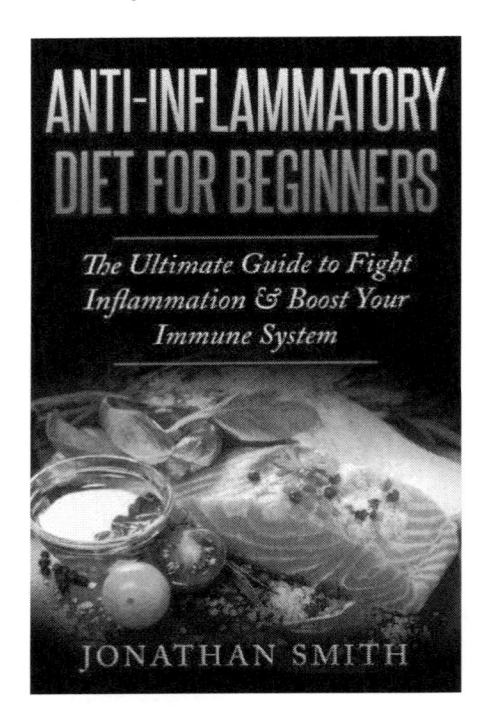

More books from us

Visit our bookstore at: http://www.dingopublishing.com

Below is some of our favorite books:

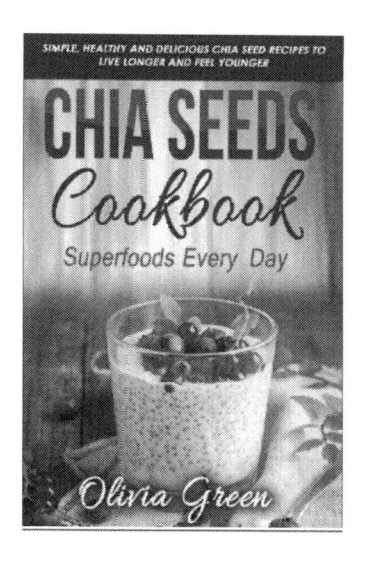

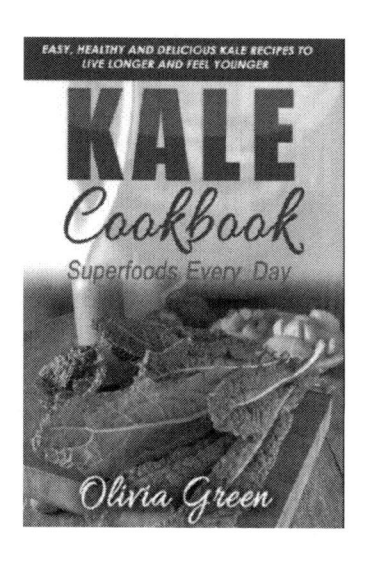

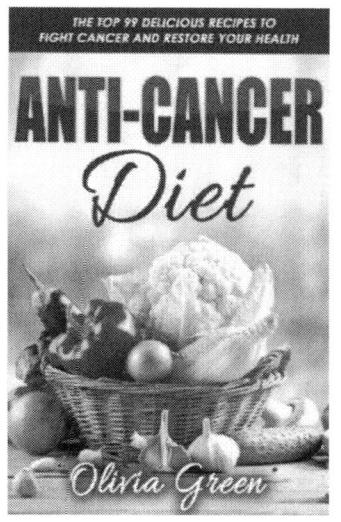

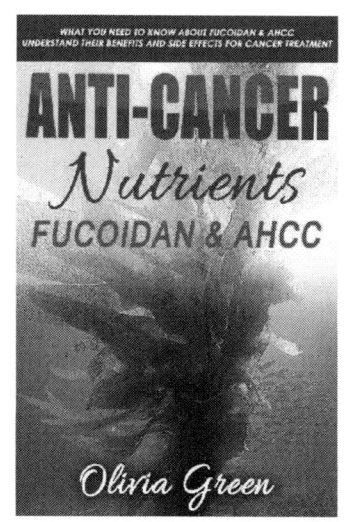

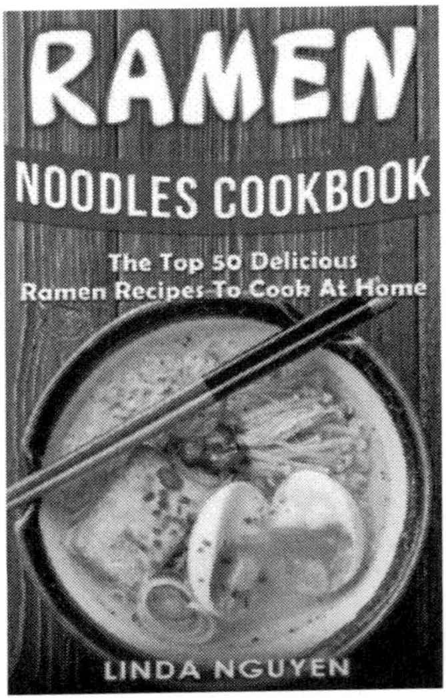
RAMEN
NOODLES COOKBOOK
The Top 50 Delicious
Ramen Recipes To Cook At Home
LINDA NGUYEN

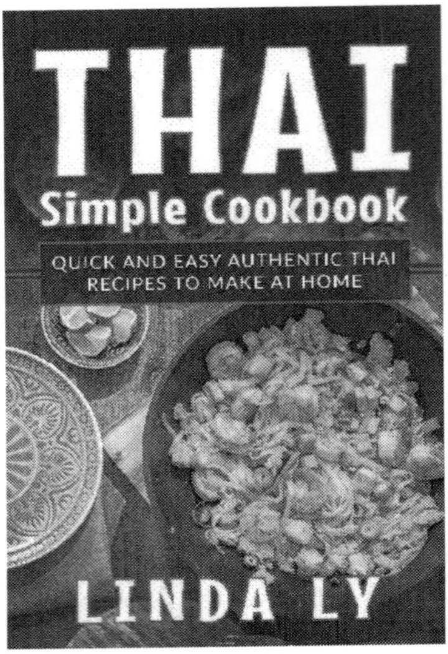
THAI
Simple Cookbook
QUICK AND EASY AUTHENTIC THAI
RECIPES TO MAKE AT HOME
LINDA LY

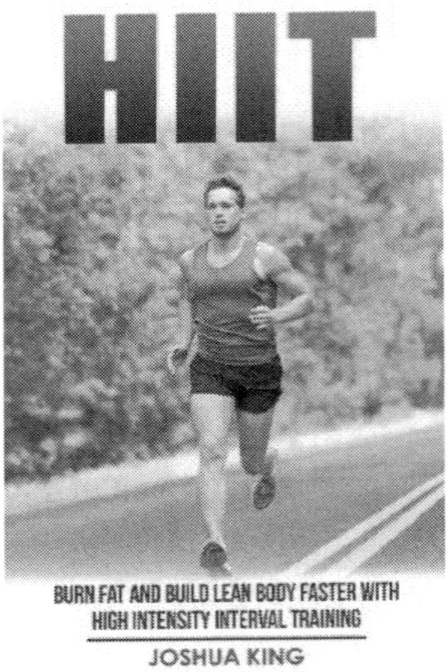
HIIT
BURN FAT AND BUILD LEAN BODY FASTER WITH
HIGH INTENSITY INTERVAL TRAINING
JOSHUA KING

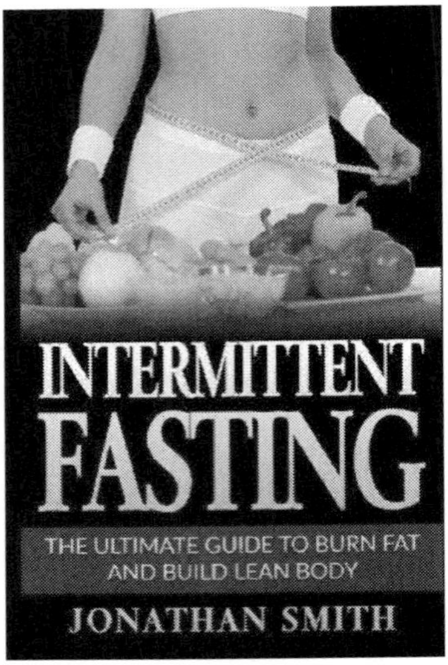
INTERMITTENT
FASTING
THE ULTIMATE GUIDE TO BURN FAT
AND BUILD LEAN BODY
JONATHAN SMITH

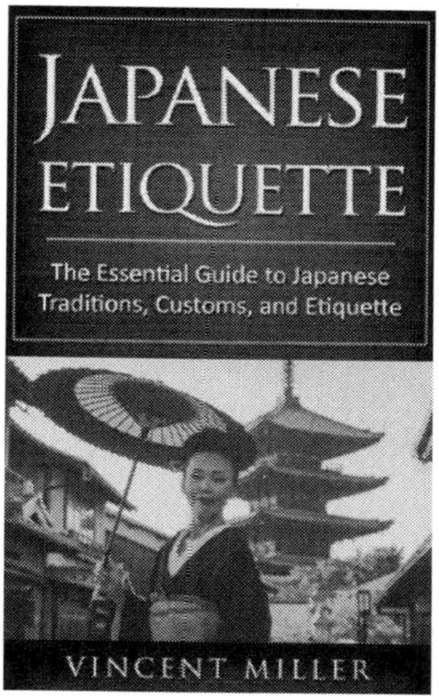
JAPANESE ETIQUETTE
The Essential Guide to Japanese Traditions, Customs, and Etiquette
VINCENT MILLER

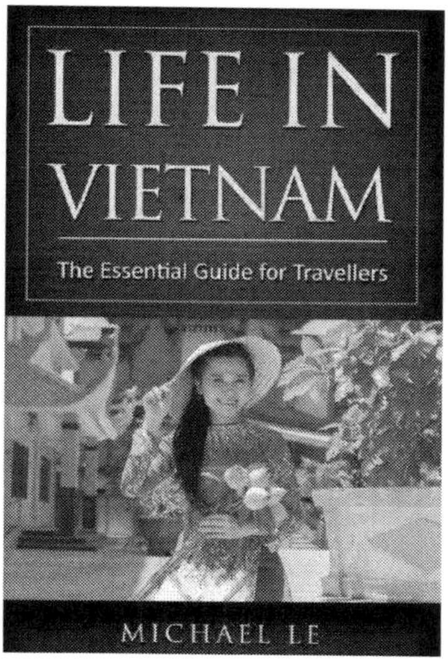
LIFE IN VIETNAM
The Essential Guide for Travellers
MICHAEL LE

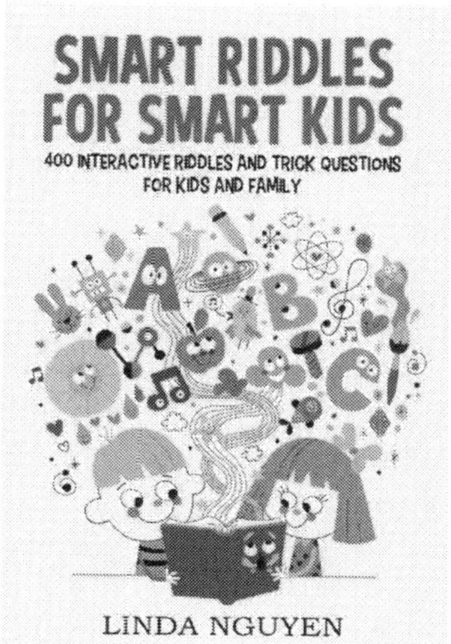
SMART RIDDLES FOR SMART KIDS
400 INTERACTIVE RIDDLES AND TRICK QUESTIONS FOR KIDS AND FAMILY
LINDA NGUYEN

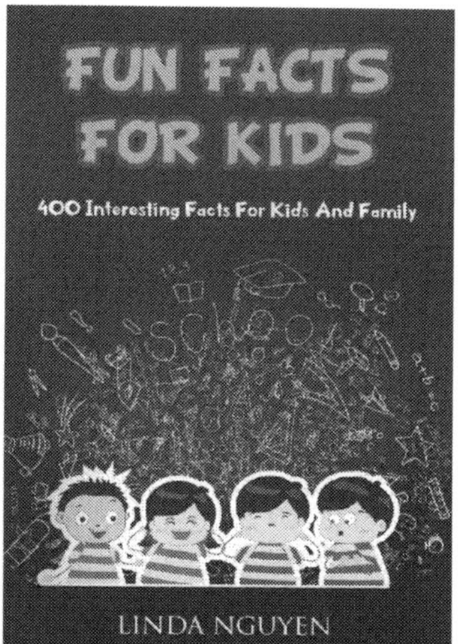
FUN FACTS FOR KIDS
400 Interesting Facts For Kids And Family
LINDA NGUYEN

Sample chapters:
'Anti-Inflammatory Diet For Beginner'
by Jonathan Smith.

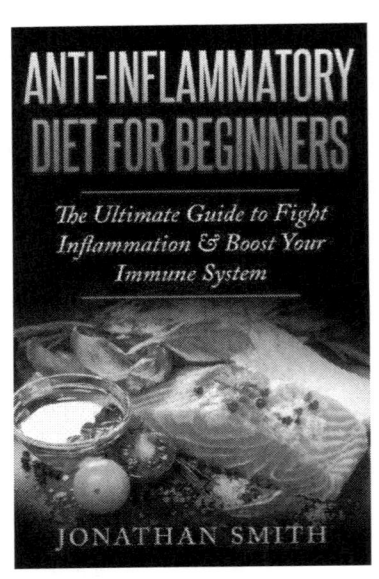

Introduction

These days, everywhere you go and every website you visit, you are going to find discussions or adverts about this or that diet program. Diets that can help you lose weight, diets that can cure cancer, and even diets that promise to increase your bank account. Some of these diets work; others are a waste of your time, energy, and financial resources. The anti-inflammatory diet is nothing like these fad diets. This revolutionary diet draws upon a simple scientific and biographical logic guaranteed to work for you regardless of your circumstances.

The anti-inflammatory diet has many innate benefits including lowering your risk of heart diseases, protecting the bones, helping you maintain a healthy weight, and increasing your body's ability to absorb nutrients from the foods you eat and the drugs you take.

This book is a comprehensive guide that shall impart upon you everything you need to know about the anti-inflammatory diet. Let's begin.

Chapter 1:
Introduction to the Anti-Inflammatory Diet

To make this book easy to read and follow, we will start by understanding inflammation and the anti-inflammatory diet.

In its simplest terms, an anti-inflammatory diet simply refers to a collection of foods that have the ability to fight off chronic inflammation in your body.

So what exactly is chronic inflammation?

Well, before we discuss that, let's start by understanding what inflammation is first.

So what is inflammation?

Inflammation is simply a term used to refer to your body's response to infection, injuries, imbalance, or irritation with the response being swelling, soreness, heat, or loss of body function. It is the body's first line of defence against bacteria, viruses and various other ailments. The goal is to 'quarantine' the area and bring about healing/relief. This is the good inflammation, as it is helpful to your body. It is often referred to as acute inflammation. However, there are times when the inflammatory process might not work as expected resulting to a cascade of activities that could ultimately result to cell and tissue damage especially if it takes place over a prolonged period. This is what's referred to as chronic inflammation. This type of inflammation has nothing to do with injuries; it is not as a result of an injury or anything related to bacteria, virus or any other microbe. And unlike acute inflammation that comes with soreness, pain, heat and swelling, chronic inflammation comes with another set of symptoms some of which include diarrhoea, skin outbreaks, congestion, dry eyes, headaches, loss of joint function and many others. This inflammation is what you need to fight using an anti-inflammatory diet because if it is not addressed early, it might result to a number of various chronic health complications that we will discuss in a while.

So how exactly does this chronic inflammation develop that would actually require a diet to undo? Here is how:

It all starts in the gut. The gut essentially has a large semi-porous lining, which tends to fluctuate depending on various chemicals that it comes into contact with. For instance, if exposed to cortisol, a hormone that is high when you are stressed, the lining becomes more permeable. The lining also becomes a lot more permeable depending on the changing levels of thyroid hormones. This increased permeability increases the likelihood of viruses, bacteria, yeast, toxins and various digested foods passing through the intestines to get into the bloodstream, a phenomenon referred to as leaky gut syndrome (LGS). The thing is, if this (the intestinal lining becomes damaged repetitively), the microvilli in the gut start getting crippled such that they cannot do their job well i.e. processing and using nutrients with some enzymes that are effective for proper digestion. This essentially makes your digestive system weaker a phenomenon that results to poor absorption of nutrients. If foreign substances find their way into the bloodstream through the wrong channels, this results to an immune response that could result to inflammation and allergic reactions. This form of inflammation can bring about different harmful complications. What's worse is that as inflammation increases, the body keeps on producing more white blood cells to fight off the foreign bodies that have found their way into the bloodstream. This can go on for a long time resulting to malfunctioning of different organs, nerves, joints, muscles, and connective tissues.

Chronic inflammation is harmful to your body and your brain. Let me explain more of this:

Your body is responsible for supplying glucose to your brain so that your brain can perform optimally. When you eat too much inflammation-causing foods, your body slows down its process of transporting glucose to the brain since it concentrates on fighting off the inflammation. Your brain then keeps asking the body for glucose since it is not getting its fill. This effect causes you to crave sugary and pro-inflammatory foods. Inflammation can also result to abnormal levels of water retention along with other problems that contribute to stubborn weight gain. This just worsens the condition and causes your inflammation to worsen. Unfortunately, majorities of dieters focused on weight loss only focus on reducing calories and fatty foods but pay very little attention to how eating pro-inflammatory foods may be contributing to an inability to lose weight quickly.

If inflammation persists, it can bring about a wide array of health complications some of which include:

- Obesity and chronic weight gain
- Lupus
- Arthritis
- Cancer
- Diabetes
- Celiac disease
- Crohn's disease
- Heart disease

So how exactly does inflammation lead to disease? That's what we will discuss next.

How Inflammation Could Lead to Diseases

It is possible to have a disease-free body, but only if you can manage to keep your body balanced. Diseases develop only when something upsets the equilibrium (balance) of the body. An abnormal composition of blood and nymph is a typical example of such imbalance. These two are responsible for supplying the tissues with nutrients and carrying away eliminated toxins, metabolic by-products and wastes from the liver and kidneys. When you consume unhealthy meals, it may affect the balance of blood and nymph in the body and lead to inadequate supply of nutrients and thus, the body would be unable to give adequate support to kidney and liver function. The consequence of this is that it exposes the body to the risks of several diseases and inflammatory conditions, which I mentioned earlier.

Food Allergies, Food Intolerance, and the Anti-Inflammatory Diet

Food allergies happen when your immune system reacts to the proteins in certain foods. Your immune system releases histamines that may cause production of throat mucous, runny nose, watery eyes, and in severe cases, diarrhea, hives, and anaphylaxis.

Your immune system's reaction to food allergies is to trigger inflammatory responses because when a food causes allergic reaction, it stimulates the production of antibodies that bind to the foods and may cross-react with the normal tissues in your body.

One of the highpoints of the anti-inflammatory diet is that it calls for the elimination of foods that promote allergies and intolerance.

How the Anti-Inflammatory Diet Works

To cure and stop incessant inflammation, you must eliminate the irritation and infection, and correct hormonal imbalance by eating specific foods while avoiding others. This would help stop the destruction of cells and hyperactive response of your immune system. When on an anti-inflammatory diet, most of the foods you shall be eating have powerful antioxidants that can help prevent and eliminate symptoms of inflammation.

For instance, anti-inflammatory foods such as avocados contain Glutathione, a powerful antioxidant. Radishes contain Indol-3-Carbinol (13C), which increases the flow of blood to injured areas. Pomegranates have polyphenols that stop the enzyme reactions the body uses to trigger inflammation. Shiitake Mushrooms are high in polyphenols that protect the liver cells from damage. Ginger has hormones that help ease inflammation pain.

We will discuss more on the foods you should eat and those you should avoid later.

In the next chapter, we shall look at the basic rules of the anti-inflammatory diet as well as how to get the best out of the diet program.

Chapter 2: Basic Rules of the Anti-Inflammatory Diet

As is the case with any diet, the anti-inflammatory diet has basic rules but as you are about to find out, these rules are very easy to follow and straightforward: no extreme rules that would leave you cravings-crazy and running back to a poor eating style after a few days.

When following this diet, there are about 11 rules you should follow:

1st: You Must Eat at Least 25 Grams of Fiber Daily

These should be whole grain fibrous foods such as oatmeal and barley, vegetables such as eggplant, onions, and okra, and fruits like blueberries and bananas. These fiber-rich foods have naturally occurring phytonutrients that help fight inflammation.

2nd: Eat at Least Nine Servings of Fruits and Vegetables Daily

A serving of fruit refers to half a cup of fruits while a serving of vegetable refers to a cup of leafy green vegetables. You could also add some herbs and spices such as ginger, cinnamon, and turmeric, foods that have strong anti-inflammatory and antioxidant properties.

3rd: Eat at Least Four Servings of Crucifers and Alliums Every Week

Crucifers refer to vegetables such as Brussels sprouts, Broccoli, mustard greens, Cabbage, and Cauliflower. Alliums refer to onions, garlic, scallions, and leek. These foods have strong anti-inflammatory properties and may even lower risks of cancer. You should eat at least four servings of these every day, and at least one clove of garlic daily.

4th: Consume Only 10% of Saturated Fat Daily

The average daily recommended calories for adults is about 2,000 calories every day. This means you have to limit your daily saturated fat caloric intake to no more than 200 calories. If you consume less than 2,000 calories daily, you have to reduce accordingly.

Saturated fats include foods like hydrogenated and partially hydrogenated oils, pork, desserts and baked goods, sausages, fried chicken and full fat diary. Saturated fats often contain toxic compounds that promote inflammation, which is why you need to eliminate these foods from your diet.

5th: Eat a Lot of Omega-3 Fatty Acid Rich Foods

Omega-3 fatty acids rich foods such as walnuts, kidney, navy and soybeans, flaxseed, sardines, salmon, herring, oysters, mackerel and anchovies are an essential part of this diet thanks to their strong anti-inflammatory properties.

6th: Eat Fish Thrice Weekly

It is important that you eat cold-water fish and low-fat fish at least three times a week because fishes are rich sources of healthy fats and can be great substitutes for saturated and unhealthy fats.

7th: Use Healthier Oils

The fact that you have to reduce your intake of some types of fat does not mean you should stop consuming all fats. You only need to reduce or even eliminate the consumption of unhealthy ones and limit your intake of healthy ones like expeller pressed canola, sunflower and safflower oil, and virgin olive oil. These oils have anti-oxidant properties that help detoxify the body.

8th: Eat Healthy Snacks at Least Twice Daily

Unlike in most diets, in this diet, you get to eat snacks as long as it is healthy. You can snack on healthy foods such Greek Yoghurt, almonds, celery sticks, pistachios, and carrots.

9th: Reduce Consumption of Processed Foods and Refined Sugars

Reducing your intake of artificial sweeteners and refined sugars can help alleviate insulin resistance and lower risks of blood pressure. It may also help reduce uric acid levels in your body. Having too much uric acid in your body may lead to gout, kidney stones, and even cancer. A high level of uric acid in the body is usually because of poor kidney function. Overloading your kidneys with pro-inflammatory foods may reduce kidney function and subsequently lead to excessive uric acid levels in the body.

Reducing your consumption of refined sugars and foods high in sodium can help reduce inflammation caused by excess uric acid within the body.

10th: Reduce Consumption of Trans Fat

Studies by the FDA reveal that foods high in trans-fat have higher levels of C-reactive protein, a biomarker for inflammation in the body. Foods like cookies and crackers, margarines, and any products with partially or fully hydrogenated oils are some of the foods with high trans-fat content.

11th: Use Fruits and Spices to Sweeten Your Meals

Instead of using sugar and harmful ingredients to sweeten your meals, use fruits that can act as natural sweeteners such as berries, apples, apricot, cinnamon, turmeric, ginger, sage, cloves, thyme, and rosemary.

Now that we have laid down the rules, the next thing we will do is to put what we've learnt into perspective i.e. what foods you should eat and what you should avoid. The next chapter has a comprehensive list of foods to consume and foods to avoid while on this diet. Consider printing out the chapter so you can use it as a reference each time you need to cook or make shopping decisions. If you do, it will not be long before you get used to the diet and can quickly decipher foods which foods you should and should not buy.

Anti-Inflammatory Diet for Beginner

By: Jonathan Smith

Find out more at:

http://dingopublishing.com/book/anti-inflammatory-diet-beginners/

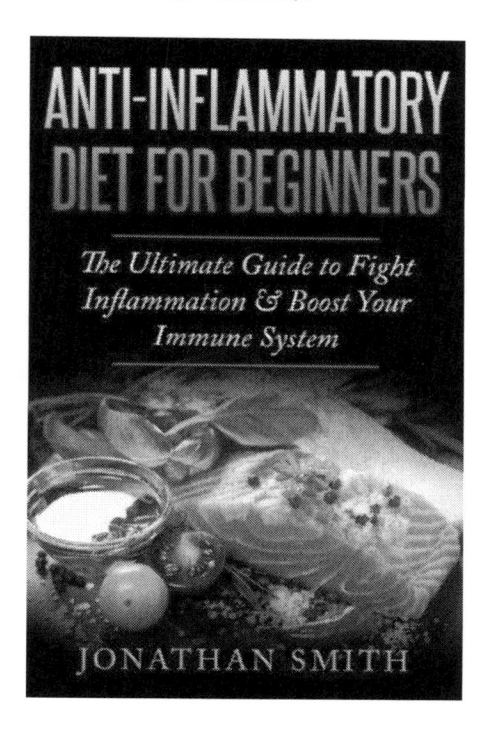

Thanks again for purchasing this book.

We hope you enjoy it

Don't forget to claim your free bonus:

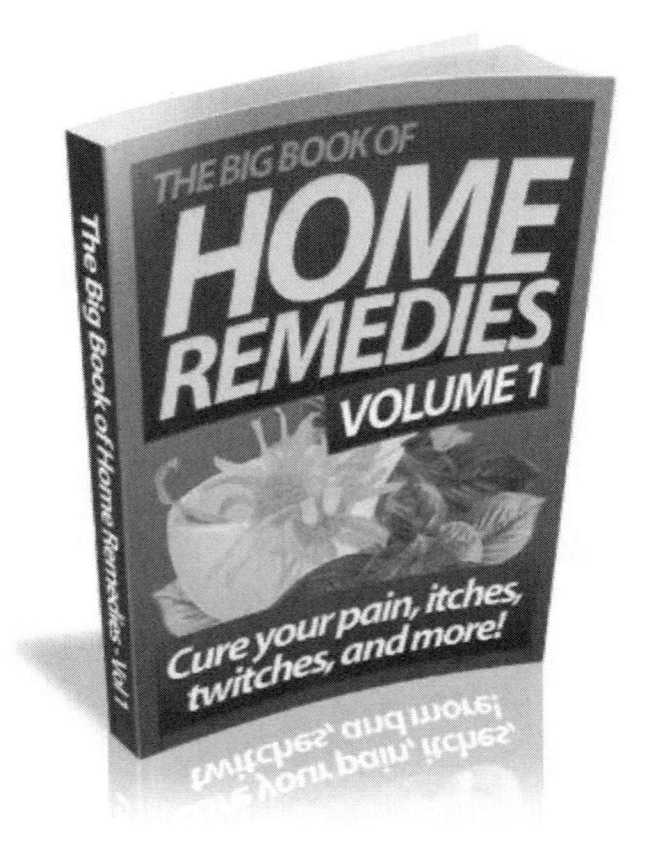

Visit this link below to claim your bonus now:

http://dingopublishing.com/heath-freebonus/

Printed in Great Britain
by Amazon